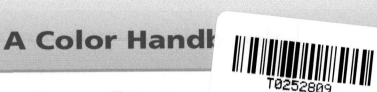

A Color Handbook

Pediatric Rheumatology

Ann Marie Reed, MD

Professor of Medicine and Pediatrics
Mayo Clinic College of Medicine
Rochester, MN, USA

Thomas G. Mason II, MD

Associate Professor of Medicine and Pediatrics
Mayo Clinic College of Medicine
Rochester, MN, USA

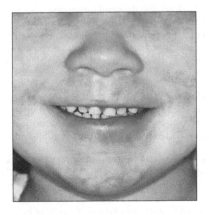

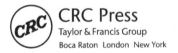

CRC Press
Taylor & Francis Group
Boca Raton London New York

CRC Press is an imprint of the
Taylor & Francis Group, an **informa** business

CRC Press
Taylor & Francis Group
6000 Broken Sound Parkway NW, Suite 300
Boca Raton, FL 33487-2742

© 2012 by Taylor & Francis Group, LLC
CRC Press is an imprint of Taylor & Francis Group, an Informa business

No claim to original U.S. Government works

ISBN-13: 978-1-84076-157-3 (pbk)

**Visit the Taylor & Francis Web site at
http://www.taylorandfrancis.com**

**and the CRC Press Web site at
http://www.crcpress.com**

A CIP catalogue record for this book is available from the British Library.
Layout: DiacriTech, India

CONTENTS

Preface 5
Acknowledgments 6

CHAPTER 1
Introduction
Thomas Mason

Assessment of the child
with rheumatic disease

Approach to children
with rheumatic disease

Inflammatory versus
non-inflammatory 8

Acute, inflammatory,
articular 8

Chronic, inflammatory,
articular 8

Chronic, inflammatory,
organ involvement 10

CHAPTER 2
Juvenile idiopathic arthritis
*Egla Rabinovich and
Angela Robinson*

Systemic arthritis 14
Oligoarthritis 21
Polyarthritis 28

CHAPTER 3
Spondyloarthropathies and reactive arthropathies
Thomas Mason

Spondyloarthropathies

Juvenile
spondyloarthropathy . . . 38

Juvenile ankylosing
spondylitis 42

Juvenile psoriatic
arthritis 48

Inflammatory bowel
disease-associated
arthropathy 50

Reactive arthropathies

Reactive arthritis 54

Post-streptococcal
arthropathies

Acute rheumatic fever 56

Post-streptococcal reactive
arthritis 58

CHAPTER 4
Lupus erythematosus
Tzielan Lee and Joyce Hsu

Systemic lupus
erythematosus 62

Mixed connective tissue
disease 76

Neonatal lupus
syndrome 80

Cutaneous lupus
erythematosus 82

CHAPTER 5
Idiopathic inflammatory myopathies
*Floranne Ernste and
Ann M Reed*

Juvenile dermatomyositis . . 88
Juvenile polymyositis 101
Postinfectious myositis . . . 103

CHAPTER 6
Vasculitis
Robert Sundel

Kawasaki disease 106

Henoch–Schönlein
pupura 109

Polyarteritis nodosa 111

ANCA-associated
vasculitides 114

Takayasu arteritis 118

Primary angiitis of
the central nervous
system 120

CHAPTER 7
Scleroderma in children
Francesco Zulian

Juvenile systemic
sclerosis 124

Juvenile localized
scleroderma 130

CHAPTER 8
Autoinflammatory diseases
Seza Özen

The monogenic
autoinflammatory diseases

Familial Mediterranean
fever 140

Cold-induced
autoinflammatory
syndrome 1
(CIAS1-pathies) – the
cryopyrin-associated
periodic fever
syndromes 144

Hyperimmunoglobulinemia D
with periodic fever
syndrome 146

Tumor necrosis factor
receptor-associated
periodic syndrome 148

Other monogenic
autoinflammatory
syndromes

Pyogenic sterile arthritis,
pyoderma gangrenosum,
and acne syndrome 150

Early onset sarcoidosis
(sporadic granulomatous
arthritis), Blau syndrome
(familial granulomatous
arthritis), and Crohn
disease 150

Autoinflammatory
syndromes that are not
monogenic/
autoinflammatory
diseases with complex
genetic traits 154

References 155
Abbreviations 169
Index 171

Pediatric rheumatology is an evolving subspecialty of pediatrics. In 1992, pediatric rheumatology subspecialty certification was offered by the American Board of Pediatrics. With advances in basic science and clinical investigation and collaboration, newer illnesses such as the autoinflammatory syndromes have been added to the pediatric rheumatology repertoire. Advances in the treatments of adult rheumatic diseases are being translated to children with comparable conditions. Pediatric rheumatology is an ever-expanding field.

Children with rheumatic diseases frequently present with primarily musculoskeletal issues but may also present with multiple organ involvement. This diversity requires that providers caring for children with rheumatic disease have a well-developed set of clinical skills. These include general pediatrics as well as familiarity with concepts about immunology, musculoskeletal medicine, and the management of chronic diseases.

This book is formatted primarily based on the most frequently recognized symptom complexes in children with rheumatic diseases. The initial chapters focus on primarily musculoskeletal issues and subsequent chapters focus on chronic autoimmune diseases that may have multiorgan involvement. We hope that you find this handbook useful to your clinical practice and a tool with which better to assess children with potential rheumatic disease.

ACKNOWLEDGMENTS

We would like to thank the chapter authors for all their time and hard work that will allow improvement of the identification of pediatric rheumatic conditions. Further, we thank all the patients who have allowed us to use their images and understand the need for early identification of these conditions. We give special thanks to Laurie Metag for her assistance in editing the text.

Introduction

- **Assessment of the child with rheumatic disease**

- **Approach to children with rheumatic disease**

ASSESSMENT OF THE CHILD WITH RHEUMATIC DISEASE

Rheumatologic diseases in general, and particularly in children, are relatively uncommon. The most common rheumatologic diagnosis for children is probably juvenile arthritis, which has a prevalence of close to 1–2:1000 children. This is similar to the prevalence of childhood diabetes and epilepsy but significantly less common than that of childhood asthma.

Frequently the differential diagnosis in these cases is quite broad. Not surprisingly, with the rarity of rheumatic disease in children, the diagnosis is often arrived at after an extensive workup for other causes. Making the diagnosis of a rheumatic disease sometimes is challenging to the clinician. Other times it is quite obvious when there is a very large swollen joint, antalgic gait, and so on.

The timeliness of arriving at a diagnosis for rheumatic disease in a child is critical. Recognition of patterns of clinical signs and symptoms is the key to making an accurate assessment as well as having a foundation to guide therapy. In the following chapters you will find descriptions of the various childhood rheumatic conditions.

The impact of the sequelae of these conditions can be profound. Certainly life- and organ-threatening consequences are occasionally seen in patients with vasculitis or connective tissue diseases. Pain, suffering, and loss of function are frequently seen in children with inflammatory arthritic conditions such as juvenile arthritis and the spondyloarthropathies. Also the consequences of treatment must be carefully considered when embarking on therapy.

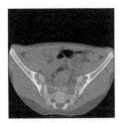 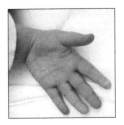 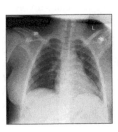 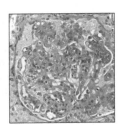

APPROACH TO CHILDREN WITH RHEUMATIC DISEASE

Inflammatory versus non-inflammatory

In sorting out symptoms, it is important to take a careful medical history although such diseases may be intermittent, with periods of inactivity. Because conditions that have an inflammatory etiology have the potential for the highest risk for damage and disability, clinical priority is given to these conditions. Inflammatory features of conditions affecting the musculoskeletal system include joint swelling, joint redness, and joint warmth in addition to joint pain and tenderness. Typically the pain is worse in the morning and gets better as the day goes on. It is helped by activity and frequently associated with stiffness.

Non-articular signs and symptoms include fevers, weight loss, chills, or night sweats. Signs and symptoms of organ dysfunction such as weakness, dyspnea, edema, and rash are clinical clues to an inflammatory extra-articular process.

Conversely, the absence of these findings as well as weight gain, and difficulty with sleep, point to a potentially non-inflammatory etiology. Chronic pain syndromes and fibromyalgia are examples of conditions that may appear to be rheumatic in nature but are not.

Based on whether the primary symptom(s) (joint pain, rash, hematuria, and so on) is (are) chronic and the history and physical examination demonstrate an inflammatory/non-inflammatory pattern, an algorithmic approach to the diagnosis of rheumatic diseases in children can be utilized.

Acute, inflammatory, articular

Almost all of the pediatric rheumatology conditions are chronic. However, clinicians involved in the evaluation of children need to be competent in evaluating acute musculoskeletal problems as well. One of these is acute monoarthritis. While the differential diagnosis includes traumatic arthropathies, the strongest consideration needs to be given to infectious causes. Septic arthritis or adjacent osteomyelitis needs to be strongly considered in any child with an acute monoarthritis with or without fever. This is a medical emergency and needs to be evaluated appropriately in a timely fashion. Infection-related arthropathies are not reviewed in this atlas.

Acute organ dysfunction such as renal insufficiency, and pulmonary dysfunction is rarely attributable to rheumatic conditions in an undiagnosed child. But, a number of the pediatric rheumatic conditions can have organ dysfunction as part of the clinical course of their illness.

Chronic, inflammatory, articular

If a child presents with chronic symptoms and the symptoms are primarily referable to the musculoskeletal system such as pain, swelling, morning stiffness, limp then the differential diagnosis includes two categories of conditions. One of these is juvenile idiopathic arthritis (JIA) and the other is spondyloarthropathies. JIA is discussed in Chapter 2 and it is contrasted with spondyloarthropathies, which are well described in Chapter 3. Subtypes of JIA have characteristic patterns of joint involvement and extra-articular manifestations including autoantibodies and inflammatory eye disease. Spondyloarthropathies have a characteristic pattern of joint involvement which includes enthesitis (also seen in some forms of JIA) and involvement in the spine as well as association with HLA-B27. An example of joint swelling associated with juvenile rheumatoid arthritis (JRA) is shown (**1**). Evidence of early radiographic change in the sacroiliac joints in a patient with spondyloarthropathy is also shown (**2**).

The most important part of the evaluation of patients with inflammatory joint disease is a careful medical history. Features of the onset, course, and duration of the symptoms is very important. Exclusion of other causes of joint pain and swelling are important as well such as those related to infectious causes. On physical examination, careful inspection and palpation of the joints are important in addition to a static and dynamic exam. Watching the child move the joint as well as the examiner moving the joint and moving the joint against resistance are important to discern the specific nature of the symptoms referable to a joint. In addition to these techniques for peripheral joints, techniques to examine the spine are outlined in the Chapter 3.

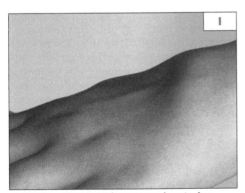

1 Wrist synovitis with cyst in polyarticular arthritis.

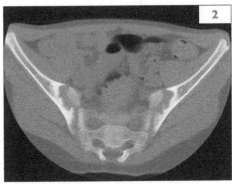

2 Scalloping of the sacroiliac joints in a 6 year old with spondyloarthropathy, severe back pain, and antalgic gait.

These patients may have evidence of inflammatory response in their blood with anemia, thrombocytosis, or leukocytosis. Acute-phase reactants such as CRP and sedimentation rate may be elevated. Some may also have autoantibodies such as RF.

In some conditions with chronic inflammatory joint symptoms, uveitis may also be seen.. The uveitis may asymptomatic (posterior) or symptomatic (anterior) as shown (3).

To summarize, patients who have chronic inflammatory symptoms referable primarily to the musculoskeletal system and confirmatory findings on X-ray (4) are likely to have JRA or spondyloarthropathy. Laboratory studies can help verify the diagnosis and give prognostic information

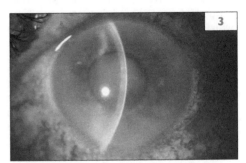

3 Red painful eye from anterior uveitis.

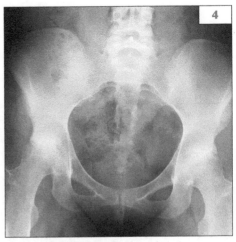

4 Hip arthritis with joint space loss in polyarticular arthritis.

Chronic, inflammatory, organ involvement

The next group of children with rheumatic diseases and inflammatory symptoms may have evidence of organ involvement apart from the musculoskeletal system. Examples of these include skin involvement with rashes from vasculitis (**5**) or vasospasm (**6**), or evidence of other organ involvement such as pleurisy (**7**), evidence of glomerulonephritis (**8**).

Since rheumatic diseases can affect any organ system, a very detailed history and a comprehensive physical exam are required to assess these patients. Unlike other subspecialties, patients may present with symptoms of any organ system so there are no characteristic historical or physical findings that would exclude a rheumatic condition. As with children with inflammatory joint symptoms, assessment of the duration and onset of the symptoms, things that make the symptoms worse or better, and interventions that have been done are important to note. A complete review of systems is also required.

On physical exam, characteristic findings such as a malar rash, painless mucositis, diminished breath sounds, edema, evidence of neurologic compromise, vasculitic rashes, and musculoskeletal weakness may be present and noted.

In these children, laboratory assessment is very important. They are necessary to assess the degree of organ damage. For example, a chest radiograph and perhaps pulmonary function studies would be required to assess chest pain or shortness of breath. Urinalysis, serum creatinine, and potentially renal biopsy for evidence to assess the cause of renal insufficiency might be needed as well. The degree of inflammation on blood tests is assessed as it is in inflammatory arthritis. The presence of autoantibodies is important as well.

To summarize, pediatric rheumatic diseases are uncommon and it often takes an astute clinician to make the diagnosis. Patterns of presentation include chronic illness that has inflammatory features. If the predominant clinical pattern is that of musculoskeletal involvement, the likely diagnostic categories include JIA and spondyloarthropathy. If organ involvement predominates, with or without musculoskeletal symptoms, then consideration of a vasculitis or connective tissue disease would be likely. My algorithm for connective tissue diseases is as shown (**9**).

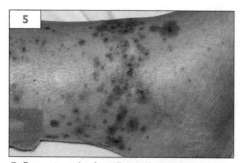

5 Purpuric rash of small vessel vasculitis.

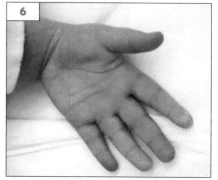

6 Vasospasm in connective tissue disease.

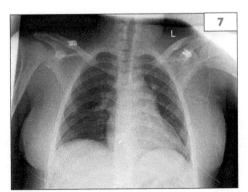

7 Pleural effusion in systemic lupus erythematosus and acute pericarditis.

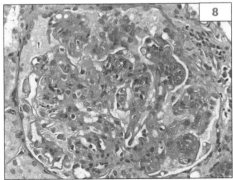

8 Glomerulonephritis in systemic lupus erythematosus.

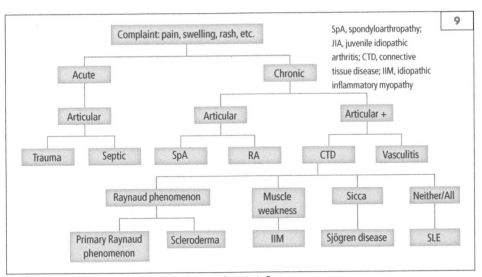

9 A rheumatologic approach to categorizing chronic inflammatory symptoms.

Juvenile idiopathic arthritis

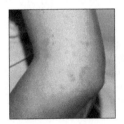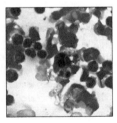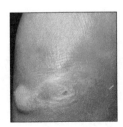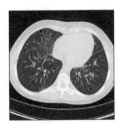

Juvenile idiopathic arthritis (JIA) is one of the most common pediatric rheumatic diseases. It is estimated that 300,000 children in the United States have arthritis, and 100,000 likely have some form of JIA (Sacks *et al.* 2007). Worldwide, the reported incidence has varied from 2 per 100,000 to 20 per 100,000 (Cassidy *et al.* 2005). True incidence is difficult to measure given the inherent difficulties in case ascertainment. Inflammatory arthritis has been described in all races and geographic areas. JIA comprises of different disease subtypes with heterogeneous phenotypic characteristics. Classification has been achieved by recognizing common clinical characteristics with the exclusion of potential mimics, and as such has been a source of debate through the years. For the purposes of this handbook, we will use the International League of Associations for Rheumatology (ILAR) criteria of classification. In general, juvenile arthritis is defined by intra-articular swelling, or the presence of two or more of the following signs: limitation in range of motion (ROM), tenderness or pain on motion, and increased heat that persists for longer than 6 weeks (Cassidy *et al.* 2005).

An international consensus conference was convened in 1997 to agree on nomenclature. The American College of Rheumatology (ACR) classification criteria are currently the only ones with corresponding ICD-9 codes in the United States. The three most widely used criteria, the ILAR classification, the ACR, and the European League Against Rheumatism (EULAR), are compared (*Table 1*) (Brewer *et al.* 1972, European League Against Rheumatism 1977, Petty *et al.* 1997). The ILAR classification includes the HLA-B27-associated spondyloarthropathies and psoriatic arthritis, subtypes categorized separately by the ACR criteria and covered in a different chapter in this handbook.

Systemic arthritis

DEFINITION
Systemic arthritis is a multisystemic inflammatory disease of which arthritis is only one of the multiple manifestations. It is characterized by the presence of arthritis and documented quotidian fever for at least 2 weeks plus at least one of the following: typical rash, generalized lymphadenopathy, hepatosplenomegaly, or serositis. Patients who fit the criteria for psoriatic arthritis, enthesitis-related arthritis, or other forms of arthritis are excluded from this category.

EPIDEMIOLOGY AND ETIOLOGY
Systemic juvenile arthritis was first described in 12 children from England by George Frederic Still in 1897. In North America and Europe systemic arthritis is one of the less-common forms of chronic arthritis, accounting for 10–20% of children seen in rheumatology clinics (Schneider & Laxer 1998, Woo 2006, Woo & Wedderburn 1998). There is no clear peak of onset as it can manifest in early childhood, adolescence, or during the adult years (then called adult-onset Still disease). Children of both genders are equally affected. It is uncertain as to whether there is seasonal variation in incidence. Recent research has indicated that these patients have high circulating levels of IL-1 and IL-6. IL-1 and IL-6 antagonists have been used clinically with improvement in some children with systemic arthritis (Pascual *et al.* 2008, Woo *et al.* 2005).

CLINICAL HISTORY
These children are usually ill with signs and symptoms of systemic inflammation (weight loss, fatigue, anemia, thrombocytosis, and elevated inflammatory markers) which tends to predominate early in the course of systemic arthritis. Temperature can rise to 39°C on a daily or twice-daily basis (quotidian pattern) and will subside to subnormal levels (**10**). Fever is characteristically elevated in the late afternoon or evening and tends to occur with the rash. Children will appear more systemically ill during fevers. Fever must be present for at least 2 weeks to fulfill diagnostic criteria. The rash that is associated with systemic arthritis is classically discrete, with erythematous macules

Table 1
Comparison of the different classification criteria for childhood arthritis

Classification	ACR (1977)	EULAR (1977)	ILAR (1997)
Name	JRA: juvenile rheumatoid arthritis	JCA: juvenile chronic arthritis	JIA: juvenile idiopathic arthritis
Minimum duration	6 weeks	3 months	6 weeks
≤4 joints at presentation	Pauciarticular	Pauciarticular	Oligoarthritis A. Persistent B. Extended
>4 joints at presentation	Polyarticular	• Polyarticular RF negative • Juvenile rheumatoid arthritis RF positive	• Polyarticular RF negative • Polyarticular RF positive
Fever, rash, arthritis	Systemic	Systemic	Systemic
Other categories included	Exclusion of other forms	• Juvenile ankylosing spondylitis • Juvenile psoriatic arthritis	• Psoriatic arthritis • Enthesitis-related arthritis • Undifferentiated A. Fits no other category B. Fits more than one category

ACR, American College of Rheumatology; EULAR, European League Against Rheumatism; ILAR, International League of Associations for Rheumatology (see text for references).

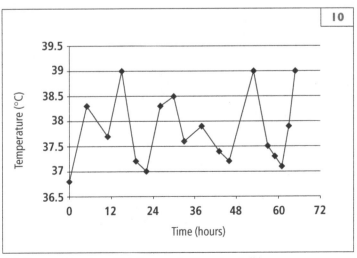

10 Fever pattern in a child diagnosed with systemic JIA.

2–5 mm in size (**11**). It is typically described as salmon-pink in color, migratory, and evanescent. It is most often found on the trunk and proximal extremities, but may develop on acral surfaces. Köbner phenomenon is often present (**12**), and it may be intensely pruritic in up to 10% of patients. Arthritis is often present initially, but may take weeks or months to manifest. Systemic JIA cannot be diagnosed without the presence of arthritis.

PHYSICAL EXAMINATION

Physical examination findings may include arthritis, tenosynovitis, fever, rash, lymphadenopathy and hepatosplenomegaly. The child may exhibit signs of cardiac or pleuropulmonary disease. Arthritis varies in manifestation, but is typically symmetric, starting in a few joints and progressing to a polyarticular course. It may present in any number of joints, and typically includes knees, wrists, and ankles. Cervical spine, hip, and TMJ disease may be present. In a minority of children, the arthritis is extremely resistant to treatment and results in an aggressively destructive course (**13, 14**). Tenosynovitis, present in 10% of children, may be seen in the extensor tendon sheaths on the dorsum of the hand (**15**), foot, and around the peroneus longus and brevis tendons of the ankle. Splenomegaly and lymphadenopathy are commonly seen, with hepatomegaly seen less commonly.

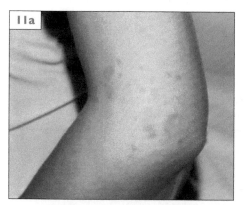

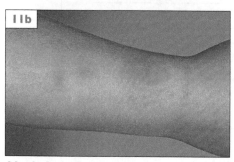

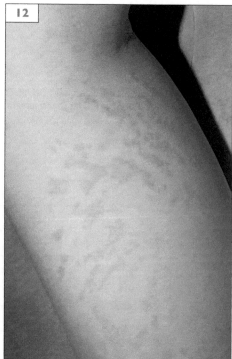

11a, b Rash of systemic JIA.

12 Systemic JIA rash exhibiting Köbner phenomenon. Note the linear distribution of the rash consistent with the history of the child scratching the involved area.

13 Radiographs of destructive hand arthritis in a child with unremitting systemic arthritis.

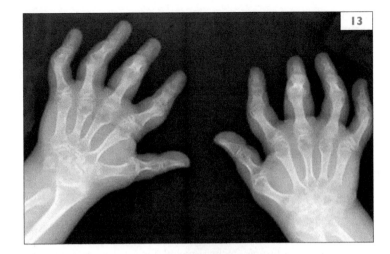

14 Cervical spine in a child with severe systemic JIA with fusion of multiple posterior facets allowing motion only at C5–6. Radiograph on left is at full extension, and on right at full flexion.

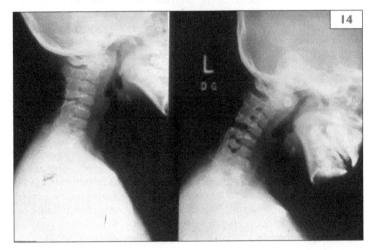

15 Tenosynovitis in the extensor tendons of the fingers, most marked in the right second, third, and fifth, and left second, third, and fourth digits.

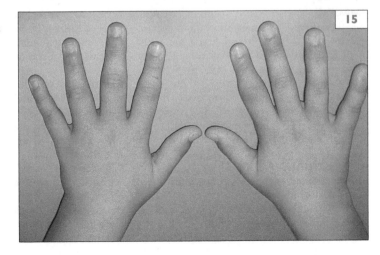

The lymphadenopathy may be marked and symmetric. Serositis may be prominent, including pericardial and pleural effusions (16). Cardiac manifestations may include myocarditis, pericarditis, and rarely endocarditis and coronary arteritis.

LABORATORY

There is no specific laboratory test for the diagnosis of systemic JIA. Laboratory markers of inflammation are typically markedly elevated (*Table 2*). White blood cell count may be in excess of 30,000 cells/mm^3 with a predominance of neutrophils. Platelets are usually elevated as well, although rarely thrombocytopenia may be present in the early stages, raising questions about concurrent or alternative conditions. A normocytic hypochromic anemia, typical for chronic disease, is seen. Sedimentation rates are characteristically high except when associated with macrophage activation syndrome, where the ESR falls to normal and is typically accompanied by cytopenias. CRP and ferritin levels are also elevated. Elevated IgG may be found, but the presence of autoantibodies such as RF and ANA is atypical. Synovial fluid analysis usually reflects inflammation with white cells in the range 10,000–40,000/mm^3. Biopsy of the rash will reveal minimal perivascular infiltration of mononuclear cells around capillaries and venules in the subdermal tissues. If there is any concern for macrophage activation syndrome or malignancy, bone marrow biopsy should be performed to evaluate for lymphoblasts or hemophagocytosis.

IMAGING

Serial radiographs may show joint space narrowing, erosions, growth arrest lines, and joint destruction. MRI and bone scan (17) may show ongoing inflammation in joints. Echocardiogram should be performed if there is any concern for pericarditis, coronary artery abnormalities, or myocarditis. If malignancy is suspected, a CT scan of the chest, abdomen, and pelvis should be considered.

DIFFERENTIAL DIAGNOSIS

At presentation systemic JIA can resemble infection, malignancy, inflammatory bowel disease (IBD), vasculitis, other connective tissue diseases, or one of the periodic fever syndromes. If corticosteroids are to be used for treatment, consider-ation of a bone marrow examination should be entertained before initiation of corticosteroids. Infections such as septicemia, acute rheumatic fever, Epstein–Barr virus, *Bartonella* sp., bacterial endocarditis, brucellosis, and Lyme disease should be considered. Malignancies such as leukemia and lymphoma may present like systemic arthritis with rash, fever, arthralgias or arthritis, and anemia. Unlike JIA, the fevers of infection and malignancy do not follow the quotidian pattern. Macrophage activation syndrome may be on a spectrum with hemo-phagocytic lymphohistiocytosis (HLH).

PROGNOSIS

Acute manifestations such as fever and rash are variable in duration, lasting from months to years, and may recur with disease flares. Approximately 50% of children with systemic arthritis recover completely, while the other half may show progressive arthritis with eventual chronic disability. In a series of patients from Cincinnati, 48% still had active arthritis 10 years later (Wallace & Levinson 1991). In a multi-center trial of 47 patients with systemic-onset JRA, there was a 37% probability of remission in 10 years (Oen *et al.* 2003). Predictors for prolonged disease and erosive arthritis include the presence of rash and fever 6 months into the disease course associated with a platelet count over 600×10^9 per liter. (Spiegel *et al.* 2000). Early studies showed a death rate of up to 14% (Stoeber 1981), but this is now thought to be much lower. Deaths in Europe were commonly due to amyloidosis; in the United States, deaths were more commonly associated with infections after corticosteroids. Macrophage activation remains a cause of mortality in these children. Unlike other forms of JIA, uveitis is generally not associated with systemic arthritis.

MANAGEMENT

Many of these children are hospitalized at diagnosis for systemic symptoms of illness and evaluation for possible sepsis or malignancy. These children rarely respond to NSAIDs alone, but these are used for fever and pain relief. Children with systemic JIA may have increased sensitivity to the hepatoxicity of NSAIDs, especially aspirin. If the diagnosis is certain with no concern for possible malignancy, glucocorti-coids may help with systemic manifestations and arthritis. Pulse methylprednisolone may be used

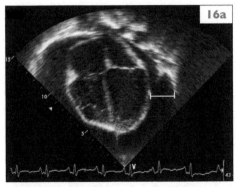

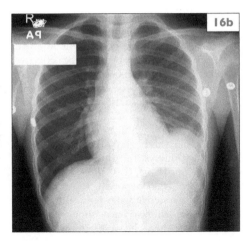

16a, b Echocardiogram showing a large pericardial effusion (white line) in a child with systemic JIA (**16a**); chest radiograph showing pleural effusion and mild mediastinal shift to the right (**16b**).

Table 2
Laboratory findings in systemic arthritis

Laboratory test	Typical result
WBC	Elevated (20,000–60,000)
Platelets	Elevated
Hemoglobin	Decreased (normocytic, hypochromic)
ESR	Markedly elevated
CRP	Elevated
Ferritin	Markedly elevated
Serum IgG	Elevated
RF, ANA	Usually negative

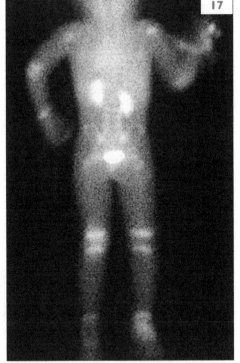

17 Bone scan of systemic JIA showing abnormal bone tracer uptake in the left knee, right ankle, right midfoot, and possibly the left radial wrist and upper cervical spine.

initially (30 mg/kg daily intravenously), with a lower daily dose of prednisone. Methotrexate has been used as a DMARD with some improvement. Anti-TNF therapy may be effective; however, there seems to be a higher proportion of non-responders to anti-TNF therapy compared with other subtypes of JIA (Carrasco *et al.* 2004, Quartier *et al.* 2003). New trials are under way for the evaluation of agents that disrupt IL-1 and IL-6/IL-6R dependent signaling pathways for therapy of systemic arthritis as anti-IL-1β, IL-1 TRAP, IL-1RA, and IL-6R have been reported to dramatically improve the systemic symptoms of the disease (18). Initial studies have showed marked response in children who were steroid dependent or resistant to other therapies (Pascual *et al.* 2008, Schneider & Laxer 1998).

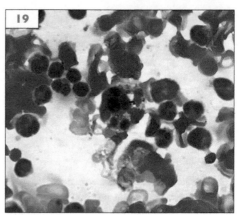

19 Bone marrow smear from a child with systemic JIA showing hemophagocytosis.

COMPLICATIONS

Complications of systemic arthritis include macrophage activation syndrome (MAS), pulmonary hypertension, cardiac anomalies, chronic deforming arthritis, and side effects due to medication toxicity. Of these MAS is most noteworthy. MAS is a macrophage-related disorder that involves dysregulation of mature macrophages, which results in fever, pancytopenia, liver inflammation, disseminated intravascular coagulation, and neurologic involvement. Muscosal bleeding, pulmonary failure, and cardiac and renal involvement may occur as well. It is closely related to secondary HLH and is associated with multiple rheumatic diseases as well as infections and malignancies. Behrens *et al.* found that 53% of 15 patients with systemic JIA had evidence of occult MAS on bone marrow aspirate, while only 13% carried a clinical diagnosis of MAS (Behrens *et al.* 2007). Laboratory findings include prolonged PT and PTT, decreased sedimentation rate from hypofibrinogenemia, markedly elevated ferritin, elevated liver enzymes, elevated triglycerides, elevated lactate dehydrogenase, and hypoalbuminemia. Abnormalities in perforin expression, granzyme B expression, and low NK cell activity have been associated with this disorder (Tristano 2008). A bone marrow biopsy can be diagnostic (19). Treatment is not standardized, but commonly involves corticosteroids, cyclosporine A, etoposide, cyclophosphamide, and other chemotherapeutic agents. Etoposide is traditionally used in treatment of HLH, but cyclosporine A has

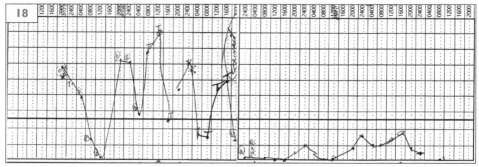

18 Fever curve in a hospitalized child with systemic JIA showing dramatic resolution of fevers with initiation of anakinra (given at 18:00 on 5/19).

been more frequently reported for treatment of MAS associated with systemic JIA. There has now been at least one case report describing the successful use of the IL-1R antagonist anakinra for the treatment of MAS.

Oligoarthritis

DEFINITION
Oligoarthritis is defined as chronic arthritis of four or fewer joints during the first 6 months of disease in a patient younger than 16 years of age. Patients who develop this in more than four joints after the first 6 months are then classified as having extended oligoarthritis.

EPIDEMIOLOGY AND ETIOLOGY
Oligoarthritis accounts for 50–60% of children with chronic arthritis in North American and European populations (Adib *et al.* 2005). Estimates of incidence are in the range 1–18/100,000 per year (Cassidy *et al.* 2005). Prevalence is estimated at 8–400 per 100,000 children (Arguedas *et al.* 1998, Danner *et al.* 2006, Manners & Bower 2002, Martinez Mengual *et al.* 2007, Oen & Cheang 1996, Pruunsild *et al.* 2007). There is a peak incidence between 2 and 4 years of age and a female:male preponderance of 3:1. Oligoarthritis developing in older boys may raise the possibility of other diagnoses such as spondyloarthropathy. It seems likely that oligoarthritis is a multigenic disease – it is seldom familial although there may be a preponderance of family members with autoimmune disease in children with oligoarthritis. HLA-A2 has been shown to be increased in children with early onset oligoarticular JRA (Murray *et al.* 1999). Oligoarthritis is strongly associated with chronic non-granulomatous uveitis.

CLINICAL HISTORY
These patients present with inflammation of four or fewer joints in the first 6 months. Oligoarthritis typically presents in the lower extremities, with knee arthritis being the most common finding (**20**). Ankles are also commonly involved (**21**). Involvement of small joints of fingers or toes is rare (presence of a finger or toe with tenosynovitis is more characteristic of psoriatic arthritis or enthesitis-related arthritis). Morning stiffness in the affected joints is common, but young children may not

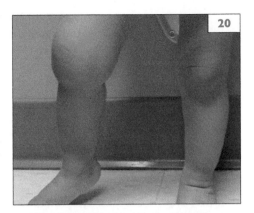

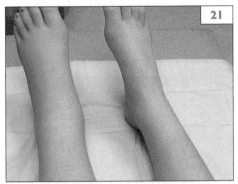

20, 21 Fifteen-month-old girl presenting with a large knee effusion associated with a flexion contracture (**20**); child with oligoarthritis and a large left ankle effusion (**21**).

be able to verbalize this symptom; parents may notice a limp in the morning that resolves by afternoon. There may be a history of the child no longer standing in the crib in the morning. Children with oligoarthritis do not usually present with extra-articular manifestations other than anterior uveitis. Uveitis may present either before or after the diagnosis of arthritis and is often asymptomatic until irreversible scarring is present. Uveitis carries a cumulative incidence of 10–15% in patients with oligoarthritis, and is more common in children with a positive ANA (Carvounis *et al.* 2006). Children may develop limb-length discrepancies or joint contractures as complications of disease. Early during the course of the disease, increased blood flow to the inflamed joint may cause increased growth of the affected limb or digit; however, continued inflammation may less commonly cause the growth plate to fuse earlier than on the opposite side, causing a foreshortened limb or digit on the affected side (**22**).

PHYSICAL EXAMINATION

The affected joint may be warm to the touch, with a ballotable fluid accumulation and restriction of range of movement. These patients do not usually complain of joint tenderness but may display joint guarding on passive range or an abnormal gait. Measurement of the length of the affected limb and examination of the back for a pelvic tilt may uncover a limb-length discrepancy (**23**). A Baker cyst may be present on posterior examination of the knee (**24**). Uveitis must be diagnosed by an ophthalmologist with a slit-lamp looking for inflammation of the anterior chamber of the eye as the uveitis is asymptomatic until scarring is present (**25**).

LABORATORY

Inflammatory markers will usually be normal. RF and anti-CCP are usually negative. ANA, present in about 50% of patients, is most helpful in predicting risk for chronic uveitis. Younger children who are ANA positive in the first few years of disease are at the most risk of uveitis and need to be screened frequently (*Table 3*). Analysis of synovial fluid should be culture negative with an increase of inflammatory cells typical of inflammatory arthritis in the range 10,000–40,000 cells/mm³. Early in the disease course, a culture of synovial fluid may be necessary to rule out infection-related arthritis.

IMAGING

Radiographs may show joint space narrowing, bony overgrowth, joint narrowing, or periarticular osteopenia (**26**), although radiographs may be normal.

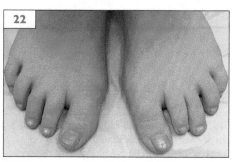

22 Twelve-year-old with history of left second toe arthritis at age 2 years now with premature closure of growth plate and shortened left toe.

Table 3
Recommended frequency of ophthalmologic screening examination in patients with juvenile rheumatoid arthritis (Cassidy *et al.* 2005)

Type	ANA	Age at onset, years	Duration of disease, years	Risk category	Eye examination frequency, months
Oligoarthritis or polyarthritis	+	≤6	≤4	High	3
	+	≤6	>4	Moderate	6
	+	≤6	>7	Low	12
	+	>6	≤4	Moderate	6
	+	>6	>4	Low	12
	−	≤6	≤4	Moderate	6
	−	≤6	>4	Low	12
	−	>6	NA	Low	12
Systemic disease	NA	NA	NA	Low	12

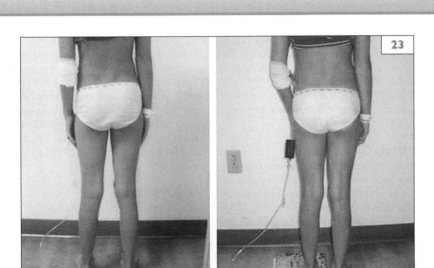

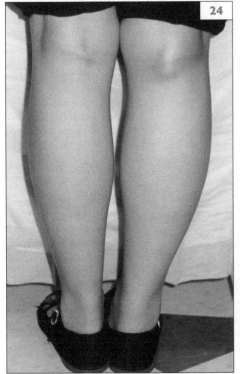

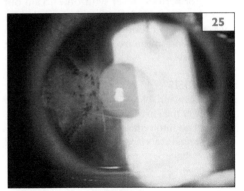

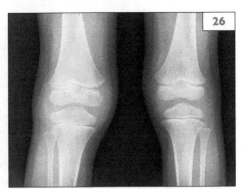

23–26 Same twelve-year-old with history of left second toe arthritis at age 2 years. Leg-length discrepancy due to JIA causing overgrowth of the right leg with pelvic tilt. A lift under the left knee corrects the pelvic tilt (courtesy of Lisa Mangino PT, DPT) (**23**); Baker cyst seen in the right posterior knee fossa (**24**); band keratopathy and iridocyclitis in a child with JIA (courtesy of Glenn Jaffe MD) (**25**); knee radiographs of a child with oligoarticular JIA with right knee involvement demonstrating epiphyseal bony overgrowth and joint effusion (**26**).

MRI with gadolinium can confirm presence of synovitis, increased intra-articular fluid and/or bone marrow edema (**27**). This may be helpful in joints that are difficult to examine clinically such as the TMJ or hips. Contrast is necessary in small joints, but not necessarily in larger joints such as the knee and hip.

DIFFERENTIAL DIAGNOSIS
Differential diagnosis includes trauma or infection, either an acute infectious arthritis due to *staphylococci*, *Streptococci*, or *Kingella kingea*, or an indolent infection such as tuberculosis (**28**). Also included in the differential is malignancy (namely bone-infiltrative cancers such as leukemia or neuroblastoma), hemophilia, or other forms of early rheumatic disease (enthesitis-related arthritis, psoriatic arthritis, sarcoidosis, systemic lupus erythematosus (SLE), or periodic fever syndrome). Pain out of proportion to physical findings, night awakenings, and abnormalities with cytopenias on the blood smear are clues to an underlying malignancy.

PROGNOSIS
Prognosis is variable. Some children continue to have fewer than five joints affected and are more likely to go into remission, although flares may occur several years later. Children with extended oligoarthritis are more likely to have progressive disease. However, serious functional disability is uncommon, and mortality is extremely rare. Uveitis activity does not correlate with severity or timing of arthritis, and may be more difficult to treat than the arthritis. JRA-associated uveitis results in decreased visual acuity in 9% of patients, with cataracts or glaucoma in 20%, and band keratopathy in 16% (**29**) (Arguedas *et al.* 1998).

MANAGEMENT
Initial management consists of NSAID therapy and consideration of an intra-articular joint injection to the involved joint(s) with corticosteroids (*Table 4* over page). Side effects of NSAIDs including gastritis and pseudoporphyria should be monitored. A physical therapy referral for passive and active stretching, along with gait training, may also be helpful. Knees and wrists that have contractures should be placed in an extension splint when sleeping (**30**). Intra-articular joint injection with triamcinolone hexacetonide is a well-tolerated, long-lasting preparation. Joint injection may be repeated up to three times per year without significant side effects, but those who continue to have ongoing disease may need methotrexate, or rarely biologic therapy. A shoe lift can be efficacious in children with significant limb-length discrepancy (>1 cm).

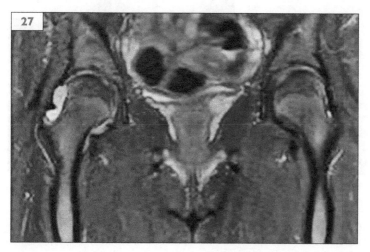

27 MRI of the hips showing effusion on right hip synovial hypertrophy and fluid on T2-weighted images.

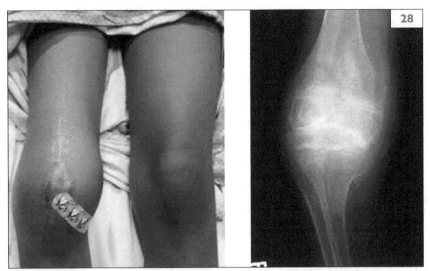

28 Child with tuberculous arthritis of the knee with corresponding radiograph demonstrating joint destruction.

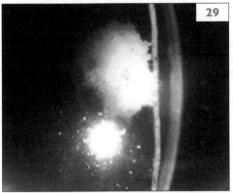

29 Severe iridocyclitis with shallow anterior chamber, posterior synechiae, and secondary cataract, seen with a slit beam from a slit-lamp (courtesy of Glenn Jaffe MD).

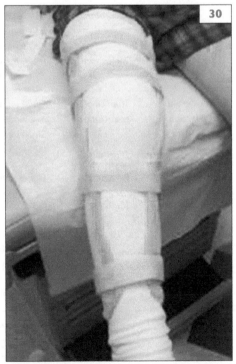

30 Leg extension splint in a child with a knee contracture that is to be worn at night to leave the leg in maximal comfortable extension (courtesy of Lisa Mangino PT, DPT).

Uveitis is managed by ophthalmologists initially with topical steroid eye drops and mydriatic agents to prevent synechiae. For uveitis unresponsive to topical drops, systemic corticosteroids, local sub-Tenon corticosteroid injections, or systemic use of methotrexate is considered. There have been multiple reports of excellent efficacy of the TNF-α-blocking antibodies (adalimumab or infliximab) for the treatment of resistant uveitis.

COMPLICATIONS

Chronic complications of oligoarthritis include limb-length discrepancy, joint contractures, periarticular osteopenia, and bony overgrowth of the affected joint. Medications may cause side effects, especially NSAID-induced pseudoporphyria. Complications related to uveitis include blindness, visual loss, cataracts, and/or glaucoma.

Table 4
Therapeutics for juvenile idiopathic arthritis

Drug class	Typical medications	Typical dosage	Indication	Side effects
NSAIDs	Naproxen (Naprosyn)	15 mg/kg orally divided twice daily	Pain relief, mild anti-inflammatory effect	Gastritis, pseudo-porphyria, renal toxicity
	Ibuprofen	40 mg/kg orally divided three times daily		
	Meloxicam	0.125 mg/kg orally daily		
Corticosteroid joint injection	Triamcinolone hexacetonide	Large joints 1–2 mg/kg Small joints 0.25–0.5 mg/kg	First-line agent for oligoarticular disease, bridging therapy	Joint infection, skin atrophy
	Betamethasone	Finger joints 0.3 mg		
Classic DMARDs	Methotrexate	0.5–1 mg/kg orally or subcutaneously weekly (10–15 mg/m^2) Give with folic acid 1 mg orally daily	Mild–moderate polyarticular arthritis	Oral ulceration, nausea, vomiting, teratogenicity, immunosuppression, hepatitis, blood count dyscrasias, concern for malignancy, GI upset, allergic rash, pancytopenia, and renal and hepatic toxicity
	Sulfasalazine	Initial: 12.5 mg/kg orally daily Maintenance: 40–50 mg/kg orally divided twice daily		

Drug class	Typical medications	Typical dosage	Indication	Side effects
	Leflunomide	10–20 mg orally daily		GI upset, hepatic toxicity, allergic rash, reversible alopecia, teratogenicity – needs washout with cholestyramine
Biologics Anti-TNF-α	Etanercept	0.8 mg/kg subcutaneously weekly	Moderate–severe polyarticular arthritis	Immunosuppression, concern for possible malignancy
	Infliximab	3–10 mg/kg intravenously every 4–8 weeks		
	Adalimumab	<30 kg: 20 mg subcutaneously every other week >30 kg: 40 mg subcutaneously every other week		
Anti-CTLA-4Ig	Abatacept	10 mg/kg intravenously every 4 weeks max 1000 mg		
Anti-CD20	Rituximab	750 mg/m^2 intravenously * 2, 2 weeks apart, max 1000 mg		
Anti-IL-1	Anakinra	1–2 mg/kg subcutaneously daily	Systemic arthritis	Immunosuppression arthritis

Polyarthritis

DEFINITION

Polyarthritis, or polyarticular JIA, is defined as chronic arthritis involving more than four joints during the first 6 months of disease in a patient younger than 16 years of age (see *Table 1*). Polyarticular JIA is further classified as RF-negative or RF positive. The RF must remain positive on two separate assays at least 3 months apart. Presence of enthesitis-related arthritis, psoriatic arthritis, and systemic arthritis is part of the exclusion criteria.

EPIDEMIOLOGY AND ETIOLOGY

Polyarthritis accounts for 30% of children with chronic arthritis. Estimates of incidence are in the range 0.29–8.9/100,000 per year (Danner *et al.* 2006, Malleson *et al.* 1996, Martinez Mengual *et al.* 2007, Moe & Rygg 1998, Pruunsild *et al.* 2007). Estimates of prevalence are in a wide range of 4.4–54.2 per 100,000 (Danner *et al.* 2006, Gäre & Fasth 1992, Martinez Mengual *et al.* 2007, Moe & Rygg 1998). Age at onset has a bimodal distribution, with an early peak between the ages of 1 and 4 years and a later peak between 6 and 12 years. RF-positive children usually present in the teenage years. Girls are affected with polyarticular arthritis more often than boys, with ratios reported of up to 4.5:1 (Moe & Rygg 1998). As with the other subtypes of JIA, the etiology is likely multifactorial and unknown. Some children may have a genetic predisposition that likely involves interaction between multiple genes. Genetic polymorphisms may be more important in RF-positive disease. Anti-CCP antibodies are less prevalent in JIA than in adult arthritis but are detectable in a significant proportion of RF-positive polyarticular JIA patients. The disease involves dysregulation of both the humoral and cell-mediated immune responses, with a pro-inflammatory cytokine profile.

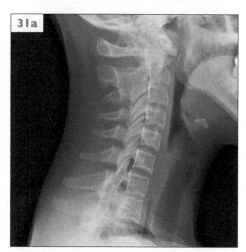

31a Cervical-spine radiograph of a child with polyarthritis showing fusion of two posterior facets at C2–3.

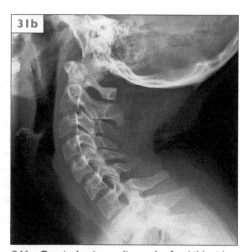

31b Cervical-spine radiograph of a child with polyarthritis showing subluxation of C2 on C3 and C3 on C4.

CLINICAL HISTORY

Polyarthritis commonly involves the large joints and tends to be symmetric. The cervical spine and TMJ are also commonly involved in this subtype (**31a, 31b, 32a, 32b**). The onset of arthritis is often subtle as a child may not complain of pain but rather may quit performing their usual functional activities. The onset is often more aggressive in those who are RF positive. A history of morning stiffness, sometimes lasting hours, or gelling after inactivity is typical. Extra-articular manifestations may include low-grade fever, anorexia with poor weight gain, and fatigue. Pericardial and pleural effusions, adenopathy, and hepatosplenomegaly may be seen, but not as

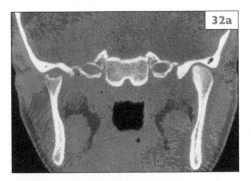

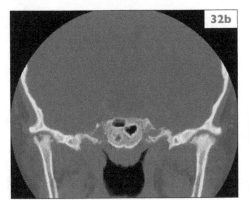

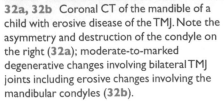

32a, 32b Coronal CT of the mandible of a child with erosive disease of the TMJ. Note the asymmetry and destruction of the condyle on the right (**32a**); moderate-to-marked degenerative changes involving bilateral TMJ joints including erosive changes involving the mandibular condyles (**32b**).

33a–c Rheumatoid nodules in a RF+ female with erosive arthritis and interstitial lung disease (**33a, b**); pseudorheumatoid nodule (**33c**).

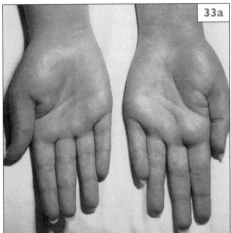

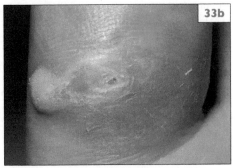

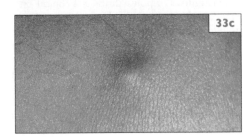

prominently as in systemic arthritis. Rheumatoid nodules occur almost exclusively in individuals with RF-positive disease (**33a–c**). A small-to-medium vessel vasculitis of the skin or internal organs may rarely occur in RF-positive polyarthritis. Other extra-articular manifestations seen in RF-positive polyarthritis, such as Felty syndrome, cardiac disease, and pulmonary involvement are rare in children compared with their adult counterparts. As in children with oligoarthritis, age and the presence of ANA are predictors for the development of uveitis and determine the frequency of necessary screening with a slit-lamp exam (see *Table 3* page 22).

PHYSICAL EXAMINATION

Inspection of the joints is helpful to assess any asymmetry. Arthritic joints have palpable fluid effusions and/or pain with restricted ROM. The involved joints may emit heat or warmth. They may be tender to palpation and sometimes have a purplish discoloration overlying, especially in the small finger joints of RF-positive patients. Arthritis is often symmetrical and can involve small joints in the hand and wrist (**34a–c**). Children may not report pain as much as adults in the clinic setting; however, on examination they may guard due to pain with ROM (Anthony & Schanberg 2007). Cervical spine involvement is often evident and is seen clinically as restricted neck extension. Auscultation of the TMJ may reveal crepitance with jaw opening and closing. Measurement of the maximal interincisal distance helps to assess and follow ROM of the TMJ. Tenosynovitis, inflammation of tendon sheaths, and synovial cysts may be present, especially in the hands (**35**). Hip involvement is not uncommon and should be evaluated by performing a complete hip ROM exam. Assessment for a leg-length discrepancy is important in children with lower extremity involvement. Patients may have an antalgic gait with a limp from involvement of the hip, knee, ankle, or feet.

LABORATORY

The diagnosis of polyarthritis is a clinical one, thus laboratory tests are only supportive. Hematologic abnormalities may be present, including leukocytosis, thrombocytosis, and anemia of chronic disease. Evidence of inflammation with elevations in ESR and CRP, along with elevated immunoglobulins, are common in polyarticular JIA. Fewer than 10% of children with JIA will have positive RF, but the presence of high titers

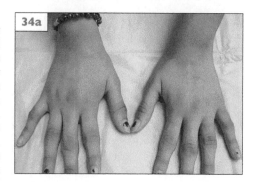

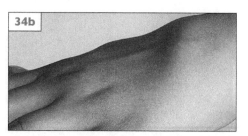

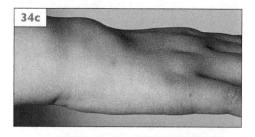

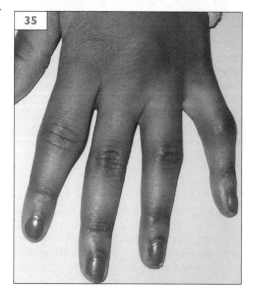

34a–c, 35 Girl with polyarthritis with involvement of wrist and fingers (**34a**); wrist swelling in a girl with polyarticular arthritis (**34b**); wrist swelling in a girl with polyarticular arthritis (**34c**); hand of girl with polyarthritis. Note the tendon sheath effusion of the second digit with fluid extending beyond the joint line, and the flexion contracture of the fifth digit (**35**).

portends a poorer prognosis (Gilliam *et al.* 2008). The presence of antibodies to CCP also suggests more aggressive disease (Gilliam *et al.* 2008). The presence of ANA indicates an elevated risk of developing uveitis (*Table 3*).

IMAGING

Plain radiographs are often normal in part because of the reduced ability to detect changes in incompletely calcified structures. Changes on radiographs may be seen early, revealing periarticular osteopenia, or decreased joint space (**36a–e**).

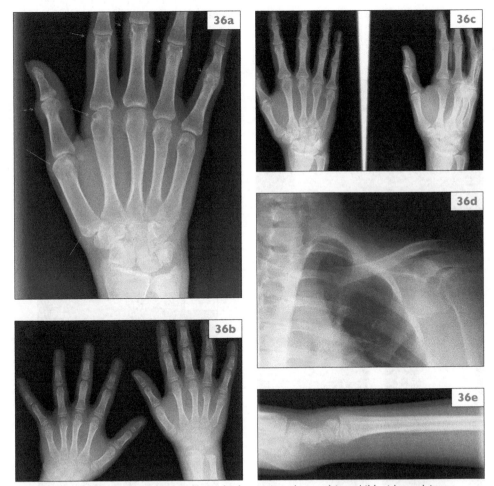

36a–e Hand radiograph demonstrating multiple erosions (arrows) in a child with recalcitrant polyarthritis (**36a**); hand radiographs at diagnosis of a 7-year-old girl with polyarthritis demonstrating periarticular osteopenia around the carpal bones (**36b, c**); shoulder joint space loss, erosions, and osteopenia in a 16-year-old girl with severe RF+ arthritis (**36d**); soft tissue swelling over wrist arthritis (**36e**).

Later bony overgrowth, bone erosions or anky-losis may occur (**37, 38**). Accelerated ossification of carpal bones may be seen in younger children (**39**). As with any form of arthritis, MRI with gadolinium can confirm the presence of synovitis, bone erosions, increased intra-articular fluid, and/or bone marrow edema (**40a, b, 41a, b, 42**). Radiographs of the hip may show structural abnormalities (**43**), but are not sensitive for demonstrating hip effusions; however, they are used to demonstrate disease pre- and post-hip replacement (**44a, 44b**)

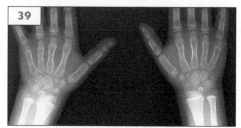

39 Hand radiographs demonstrating asymmetric and accelerated carpal maturation on involved left hand compared with non-involved right hand. There is early ossification of the ulnar styloid and larger trapezoid and scaphoid bones on the left.

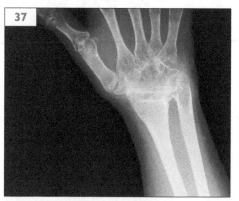

37 Ankylosis of the wrist bones in a patient with polyarticular arthritis.

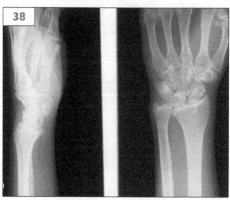

38 Hand radiograph demonstrating carpal and metacarpal–phalangeal ankylosis in a child with recalcitrant polyarthritis.

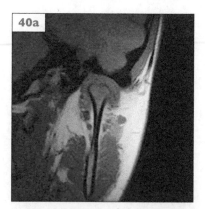

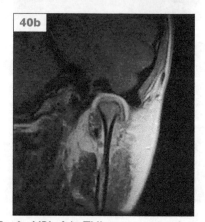

40a, b MRI of the TMJ: pre-contrast infusion showing flattening of the condyle (**40a**); post-contrast image with gadolinium showing a joint effusion of the TMJ (**40b**).

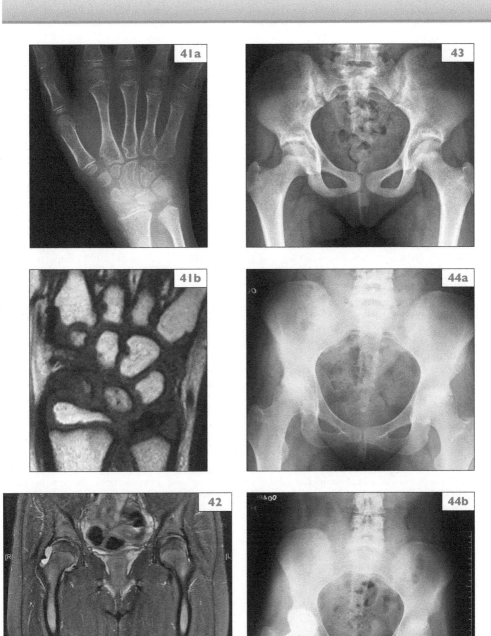

41a, b, 42 Eight year old with wrist arthritis seen on plain radiograph demonstrating erosions and crowding of the carpal bones (41a); 8 year old with wrist arthritis: contrast-enhanced MRI of the same wrist demonstrates erosions and synovial enhancement and fluid within the joint (41b); hip MRI demonstrating hip effusion on the right (42).

43, 44a, b Hip radiograph revealing flattened femoral heads from long-standing polyarthritis (43); 16 year old girl with severe RA pre hip replacement (44a); 16 year old girl with severe RA post-hip replacement (44b).

Ultrasound can be particularly helpful in evaluation of possible hip effusion (**45**). Chest imaging is warranted with concerns for arthritis-related lung disease; CT scan demonstrates ground glass throughout the lung fields and nodules (**46a, 46b**).

DIFFERENTIAL DIAGNOSIS

Differential diagnosis includes polyarthritis associated with other rheumatologic diseases, including SLE, enthesitis-related arthritis, sarcoidosis, dermatomyositis, and scleroderma. The arthritis associated with these other autoimmune diseases may be difficult to differentiate from polyarticular JIA without looking for characteristic clinical or laboratory findings (e.g. presence of double-stranded DNA antibodies indicative of lupus or rash of dermatomyositis). Infections most often cause oligoarticular arthritis, but rarely present with a polyarticular picture, such as with infections caused by *Neisseria gonorrhoeae*, acute Lyme disease, or acute rheumatic fever. Polyarthritis may be found in children with serum sickness, IBD, and sickle cell disease. Whipple disease is another rare cause of polyarticular arthritis. Malignancies may cause periarticular pain and swelling or actual joint effusions, and are included in the differential diagnosis.

PROGNOSIS

Poor predictors of outcome include delay in diagnosis, longer disease duration, persistent active disease, early development of bony erosions, and presence of subcutaneous nodules. RF seropositivity and presence of anti-CCP are also poor predictors, and these patients tend to have more aggressive disease unless aggressively treated (Gilliam *et al.* 2008, Habib *et al.* 2008, Selvaag *et al.* 2005). Overall prognosis for a life without disability is good, however, especially with the increase in number of new available medications.

MANAGEMENT

NSAIDs are used for pain relief and decrease in inflammation but alone rarely prevent joint damage (see *Table 4*). Second-line medications, including DMARDs, are often required to treat polyarthritis. Methotrexate has long been the standard therapy for polyarthritis. It is given in low-dose, weekly administration either by mouth or by subcutaneous injection (for improved absorption). Both leflunomide and sulfasalazine have been shown to be beneficial (Silverman *et al.* 2005, van Rossum *et al.* 1998). Biologic agents, specifically TNF-α inhibitors, are becoming more important in the management of polyarticular disease (Lovell *et al.* 2000, Lovell *et al.* 2008, Ruperto *et al.* 2007). Anti-TNF-α agents include etanercept, adalimumab, and infliximab. Abatacept, which blocks T-cell costimulation, has recently been approved for use in polyarticular JIA (Ruperto *et al.* 2008). Rituximab, an antibody directed toward B cells, has been shown to be effective in adult rheumatoid arthritis (Cohen *et al.* 2006). Intra-articular injections of corticosteroids can be used to treat a few recalcitrant joints, or as a bridging therapy while awaiting the effects of DMARD treatment. Systemic corticosteroids should be used sparingly, with prolonged use discouraged due to the unique side effects on the growing skeleton such as growth retardation and osteopenia. Physical therapy and occupational therapy are also important elements in the treatment of children with polyarthritis as attention needs to be paid to not only current functional status but also expected changes with growth and maturity. Children may need special school accommodation provided.

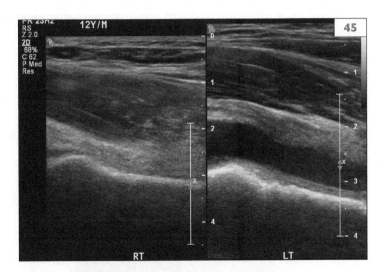

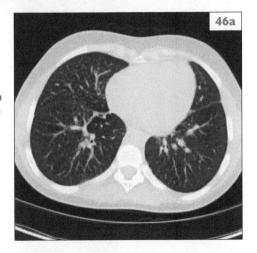

45 Ultrasound scan of bilateral hips revealing large effusion on the right.

46a, b CT chest scan of 11-year-old girl with RF+ arthritis, rheumatoid nodules, and interstitial lung disease with ground-glass appearance and pulmonary nodule.

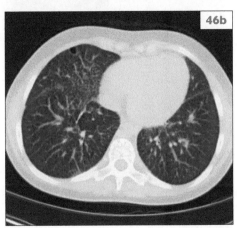

COMPLICATIONS

Chronic arthritis can lead to disturbances in growth of the involved joint, causing bony overgrowth, lengthening of an affected limb, or premature closure of growth plates and shortening of an affected limb. With chronically active disease, overall linear growth of a child may also be slowed. Chronic complications also include joint contractures with restriction in ROM, erosive changes in bone, and periarticular osteopenia (**47**, **48**). Disease of the TMJ in polyarthritis can lead to micrognathia and retrognathia. Disease of the cervical spine in polyarthritis can lead to degeneration of the vertebral bodies and cervical spine fusion, and may lead to impingement of the spinal cord (see **31a**, **31b**). Medications used to treat arthritis may also have side effects.

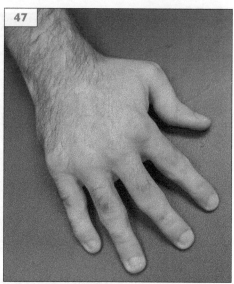

47 Hand in a 19 year old with polyarthritis. He was initially diagnosed with polyarthritis at age 3 years and now has contractures at his MCPs with subluxation at the base of his thumb. His pip contractures have been surgically corrected.

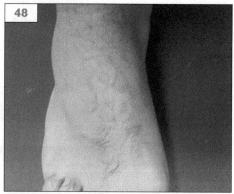

48 The same young man (as shown in **47**) demonstrating contractures of toes.

CHAPTER 3

Spondyloarthropathies and reactive arthropathies

- Spondyloarthropathies

- Reactive arthropathies

- Post-streptococcal arthropathies

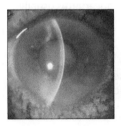
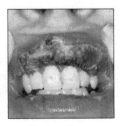
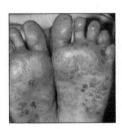
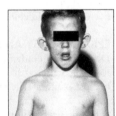

The term 'spondyloarthropathy' refers to a collection of inflammatory conditions in which both axial (spine) and appendicular (peripheral) joints are involved. Inflammation at the sites of ligamentous insertion, also know as enthesitis, is also a hallmark of these diseases. The joint involvement is primarily in the lower extremities and develops at age 16 years or younger (Gensler & Davis 2006).

Reactive arthropathies can be defined as a sterile inflammatory arthropathy temporally associated with a remote antigenic exposure. While this antigenic exposure is usually infectious, in conditions like serum sickness, a similar reactive inflammatory arthropathy can occur to non-infectious agents such as a medication. One of the challenges in writing about these conditions is the diversity in terminology that has been used in the past to describe these conditions. Several of these conditions have been labeled in alternative ways and presently could be better classified as forms of juvenile idiopathic arthritis (JIA). Examples of this include juvenile psoriatic arthritis and enthesitis-related arthritis which are subtypes of JIA in the ILAR classification system (see below). Unfortunately, much of the literature describing these conditions predates these criteria, and so the previous framework for describing these conditions is used in this chapter. An example of this approach is shown in the next section on the broad category of juvenile spondyloarthropathy.

SPONDYLOARTHROPATHIES

Juvenile spondyloarthropathy

DEFINITION
In 1991 criteria were established by the European Spondyloarthropathy Study Group (ESSG) to diagnose spondyloarthropathies in which one major criterion and one minor one are required (Dougados *et al.* 1991). These criteria are summarized (*Table 5*). The ESSG criteria have been validated in children (Prieur *et al.* 1990).

EPIDEMIOLOGY AND ETIOLOGY
Determining epidemiologic data for juvenile spondyloarthropathy (JSpA) is challenging because of plural criteria for diagnosis, lack of key clinical features at diagnosis, and the lack of confirmatory radiographic data, particularly

Table 5
Criteria for the diagnosis of spondyloarthropathy (Dougados *et al.* 1991)

Major criteria	Minor criteria
Synovitis that is asymmetric or predominantly of the lower limbs	Positive family history, which is defined as presence in first-degree or second-degree relatives psoriasis, acute uveitis, reactive arthritis, or IBD
Inflammatory spinal pain	Psoriasis diagnosed by a physician; IBD (either Crohn disease or ulcerative colitis) diagnosed by a physician and confirmed by radiographic examination or endoscopy
	Non-gonococcal urethritis or cervicitis, or acute diarrhea within 1 month before arthritis
	Buttock pain alternating between right and left gluteal areas
	Enthesopathy, defined as spontaneous pain or tenderness at the site of insertion of the Achilles tendon or plantar fascia
	Radiographic evidence of sacroiliitis by plain films

At least one major criterion and one minor criterion are needed to make diagnosis of spondyloarthropathy. Inflammatory spinal pain is defined as three of the following: at least 3 months' duration, onset before 45 years of age, insidious onset, improved by exercise, or associated with morning stiffness.

Box 1 Keys to recognizing JSpA

- Chronic, inflammatory arthritis usually oligoarticular, lower extremities
- Enthesitis
- IBP
- Anterior uveitis
- Associated disease features: nail pits, psoriatic rash, mucositis, dysuria, diarrhea, and so on.

of the axial skeleton. Estimates of the prevalence of JSpA based on inventories of patients seen at pediatric rheumatology centers suggest that from 1% to 20% of children with a specific rheumatic condition may have JSpA (Rosenberg 2000). The etiology of JSpA is largely unknown, but seems to be associated with HLA-B27 (see below).

CLINICAL HISTORY

Key clinical features of JSpA are shown (**box 1**). Since less than one-quarter of children with JSpA have axial spine pain, stiffness, or restricted motion or signs or symptoms of sacroiliitis at presentation (Rosenberg 2000), the diagnosis is often delayed. The diagnosis often rests on finding inflammatory arthritis in the lower extremities along with at least one of the minor ESSG criteria, for example knee involvement as shown (**49**).

Another prominent clinic feature of JSpA is uveitis. Anterior uveitis (**50**), which is usually associated with pain, photophobia and redness, is more associated with ankylosing spondylitis (AS) and reactive arthritis (ReA) (Paiva *et al.* 2000). Posterior uveitis (**51**) is more subtle, often painless, and even asymptomatic. In JSpA, posterior uveitis is seen more with psoriatic arthritis (PsA) and the arthropathy associated with IBD (Paiva *et al.* 2000).

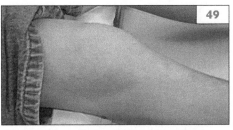

49 Right knee effusion. Notice the swelling in lateral suprapatellar pouch of the right knee. This 14-year-old boy had a bulge sign and pain on extreme knee flexion, but no antalgic gait. Oligoarthritis of the lower extremities is a frequent presentation for spondyloarthropathies.

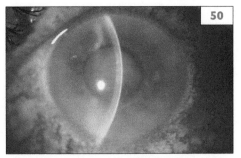

50 Acute anterior uveitis with hypopyon. Note the marked conjunctival injection and the cloudiness of the anterior chamber. These patients usually present with red eye and eye pain with photophobia (courtesy of D. C. Herman, MD, Mayo Clinic).

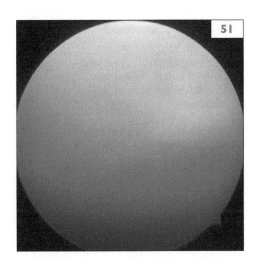

51 Severe posterior uveitis. In this funduscopic image the vitreous is so cloudy with inflammatory cells that it is difficult to make out other normal structures such as the disc, vessels, or retinal detail (courtesy of D. C. Herman, MD, Mayo Clinic).

PHYSICAL EXAMINATION

Enthesitis is a term that refers to inflammation at the sites of ligamentous insertion on to bone near a joint. Frequent areas of enthesitis in spondyloarthropathies include the insertion of the Achilles tendon (**52**) and that of the plantar fascia on the heel, and the patellar tendon insertion on the tibia. These areas are tender on exam, and may be red, warm or swollen. While joint pain, swelling, tenderness, limited ROM, and enthesitis are hallmark features of all forms of JSpA, other common distinguishing clinical features (including axial findings) will be discussed later.

LABORATORY

Routine laboratory studies such as CBC, ESR, and CRP may show evidence of an inflammatory process with elevations in the WBC, platelet count, ESR, and CRP and evidence of the anemia of chronic disease. The presence of HLA-B27 increases the odds ratio of a diagnosis of a JSpA, particularly if there is axial involvement. The prevalence of HLA-B27 is not clear in JSpA although estimates have ranged from 40% to 90% (Burgos-Vargas 2002, Rosenberg 2000). Autoantibodies are not commonly seen in JSpA.

IMAGING

Imaging of the peripheral joints may show soft tissue swelling that is apparent on clinical exam. Rarely destructive changes such as joint space narrowing or erosions may be present.

Plain radiographs of the spine are frequently normal, even in those with axial involvement of JSpA. With more sensitive imaging techniques, such as CT and MRI, the presence of inflammatory changes around the sacroiliac (SI) joints may be more apparent, for example early subtle changes in JSpA (**53**), and more dramatic SI disease (**54a, 54b**).

DIFFERENTIAL DIAGNOSIS

Since axial involvement is uncommon at the outset of JSpA, other conditions that share the clinical features of inflammatory arthritis, particularly an oligoarthritis of the lower extremities in children should be considered. One of these is enthesitis-related JIA. Children with enthesitis-related JIA may later develop a more classic spondyloarthropathy as described above. These criteria were developed in 1998 and updated in 2001 (Petty *et al.* 2004) (*Table 6*).

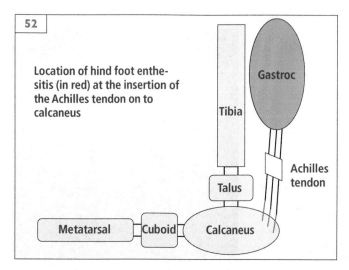

52 Enthesitis. This diagram shows (in red) the area of inflammation in enthesitis of the Achilles tendon at its insertion on the calcaneus. Gastroc, gastrocnemius muscle.

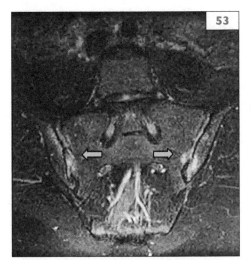

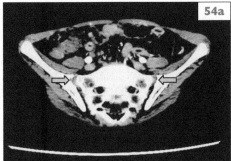

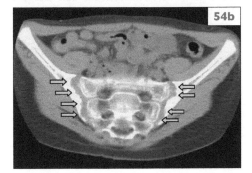

53, 54a, b Early sacroiliitis. In this T2-weighted MRI scan, subtle findings of bone marrow edema (lighter areas) adjacent to the SI joints are highlighted by arrows (**53**); CT scan of SI joints of a 6-year-old boy with bilateral gluteal pain and waddling gait who was HLA-B27 negative. There are erosions (arrows) on the sacral side anteriorly of both SI joints, more impressively on the right. The SI joints were aspirated and all cultures were negative (**54a**); CT scan of SI joints of the same boy (**54a**) 26 months later. Notice the marked increase in number of erosions (arrows) especially on the iliac side of the SI joints and the demineralization of the sacrum in spite of treatment with sulfasalazine and oral methotrexate. The child responded dramatically to etanercept therapy (**54b**).

Table 6
Criteria for the diagnosis of the enthesitis-related arthritis subgroup of juvenile idiopathic arthritis (Petty *et al.* 2004)

Diagnosis confirmed	Diagnosis confirmed	Exclusions
Arthritis *and* enthesitis	Arthritis *or* enthesitis with at least two of the following:	Dermatologist confirmed psoriasis in at least one first-degree relative
	• (+) HLA-B27	Systemic onset arthritis
	• Sacroiliac tenderness and/or inflammatory spinal pain	Positive RF
	• Family history in first-degree relative with uveitis, AS, ReA, IBD-related sacroiliitis, or enthesitis-related arthritis	
	• Anterior uveitis, acute	
	• Arthritis in a boy after age 6 years	

The other common condition with similar features is pauciarticular juvenile rheumatoid arthritis (pauci-JRA). In the US, many of these children will be initially diagnosed with pauci-JRA, reflecting the slight difference in nomenclature between JIA and JRA. There are similarities and differences between the spondyloarthropathies and pauci-JRA (*Table 7*).

PROGNOSIS
In population-based studies from Norway, children with spondyloarthropathies were a subset of children with chronic arthritis sho had a poorer outcome (Selvaag *et al*. 2005). In these studies of nearly 200 children with JRA, 7 with JSpA, and 5 with juvenile PsA (JPsA), those with JSpA and JPsA had lower levels of physical function and wellbeing, and higher levels of pain compared with the rest of the cohort (Selvaag *et al*. 2005).

MANAGEMENT
Within the management principles for chronic rheumatic diseases in general, there are particular treatment principles for JSpA (**box 2**). More specific aspects of medical management of the axial and peripheral arthritis of JSpA will be highlighted in the following sections.

COMPLICATIONS
The potential complications of the various forms of JSpA will be discussed below.

Box 2 Treatment principles for management of JSpA

- Establish correct diagnosis
- Assess pain, functional status and risk for progression and damage
- Patient/family education
- PT/OT to optimize functional status
- Medications administered after risk/benefit ratio assessment

---

Juvenile ankylosing spondylitis

DEFINITION
Juvenile ankylosing spondylitis (JAS) is defined as the diagnosis of AS before age 17 years; it may also be called juvenile- onset ankylosing spondylitis (JoAS) to contrast with adult-onset ankylosing spondylitis (AoAS) (Burgos-Vargas *et al*. 1997). The diagnosis of AS is made based on a combination of clinical and radiographic features (*Table 8*). These criteria (van der Linden *et al*. 1984) are weighted heavily to radiographic findings.

EPIDEMIOLOGY AND ETIOLOGY
The prevalence of AS is in the range of around 70–210 cases per 100,000 adults and has an incidence of between seven and nine cases per 100,000 person-years depending on the population studied (van der Linden *et al*. 2008). In patients diagnosed with AS, about 10–20% will be before age 17 years (JAS), although there are populations with higher juvenile prevalence in Mexico and Korea (Burgos-Vargas *et al*. 1996). The etiology of JAS is not known, but is also associated with HLA-B27 (see below).

CLINICAL HISTORY
Patients with JAS frequently present with non-axial symptoms and a high index of suspicion is needed to make this diagnosis. Confirmatory radiographic findings are frequently absent early in the illness. The key feature of axial involvement is inflammatory back pain (IBP). Features of IBP include stiffness, particularly in the mornings, that is helped by activity and chronicity (usually months of symptoms). Sometimes the pain will be perceived in the buttocks.

In a Korean study of nearly 100 consecutive AS cases from 1997 to 1998, patients with JAS were more likely to present with peripheral joint symptoms and less likely to present with spinal symptoms compared with adults with AS (Baek *et al*. 2002). In this study radiographic findings of ankylosis and syndesmophytes were much less in the JAS group as was limitation of spinal ROM (Baek *et al*. 2002). Similar findings were described in 150 patients with AS and 60 with JAS from India (Aggarwal *et al*. 2005).

Table 7
Comparison of clinical features of juvenile spondyloarthropathies and juvenile rheumatoid arthritis

	Pauci-JRA	JSpA
Age at onset	Preschoolers	Older
Gender	Girls	Boys
Spine involvement	No	Characteristic, but often not at diagnosis
SI involvement	No	Characteristic, but often not at diagnosis
Enthesitis	No	Characteristic
Uveitis	Chronic posterior (increased with positive ANA)	Acute anterior
Joint involvement	Oligoarthritis	Oligoarthritis
Autoantibodies	ANA	None
HLA associations	Mostly class II, multiple	Class I: B27
Other associated conditions	–	Psoriasis, IBD, GI/GU infections, oral mucositis

Table 8
Criteria for the diagnosis of ankylosing spondylitis (van der Linden *et al.* 1984)

Radiographic findings	Clinical findings
At least moderate bilateral SI changes (at least 2 on a 4-point scale)	IBP
At least severe unilateral SI changes (at least 3 on a 4-point scale)	Restricted ROM in lumbar spine in at least planes of movement
	Decreased chest expansion

At least one radiographic feature and one clinical feature are needed to make the diagnosis of AS.

PHYSICAL EXAMINATION

Inflammatory oligoarthritis, particularly in the lower extremities, and enthesitis are common features of JAS, and were discussed previously. An assessment of the ROM of the spine and the presence of SI tenderness is critical to evaluate children with JAS.

To assess SI tenderness, direct palpation is important, but may be difficult to reproduce. Compressive maneuvers such as the Patrick test may be more specific (**55**). This test is also known as the FABER maneuver (*f*lexion, *ab*duction and *e*xternal *r*otation).

To assess spine ROM, the spine is examined in three regions: cervical, thoracic, and lumbar. There are several techniques for examining each region, and an example for each follows. To assess cervical spine ROM, the wall-to-tragus measurement is helpful (**56**). To assess thoracic spine mobility, measurement of chest expansion is done (**57**). Measurement of lumbar spine ROM may be assessed by the modified Schober test (**58**).

LABORATORY

Routine laboratory studies such as CBC, ESR, and CRP may show evidence of an inflammatory process with elevations in the WBC, platelet count, ESR, and CRP and evidence of the anemia of chronic disease. Almost 90% of JAS patients are HLA-B27 positive (Baek *et al.* 2002, Gensler *et al.* 2007). Autoantibodies currently measured are most often absent in JAS.

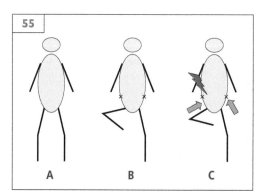

55 Patrick test. The patient, while supine on an examination table (A), is asked to flex and externally rotate a hip (B). Then pressure from the examiner is placed on the contralateral anterior iliac crest and the ipsilateral femur towards the lumbar spine (C). SI pain is usually perceived in the ipsilateral SI area. This is repeated on the opposite side to assess each SI joint.

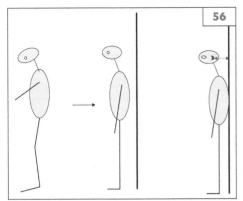

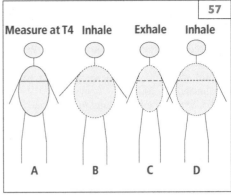

56, 57 Wall-to-tragus distance. A patient stands against a wall or stable vertical planar surface, keeping knees straight, eyes looking straight ahead, and chin parallel to floor. The patient is then asked to extend his or her neck and the distance from the posterior tragus to the wall is measured and recorded. This measurement helps assess cervical spine ROM (**56**). Chest expansion. From behind a standing (or seated) patient, a tape measure is placed around the chest at T4. The patient is asked to take a deep breath (B), and then exhale. The chest circumference is measurement at the end of exhalation and noted (C). The patient is then asked to take another deep breath (D), and the measurement of chest circumference at maximum inhalation is noted. Chest expansion is the difference in measurements at points C and D (**57**).

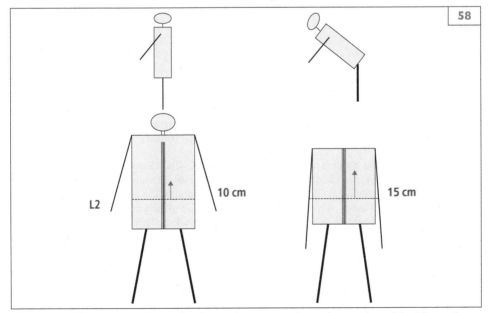

58 Modified Schober test. From behind a standing patient, the surface marker of the L2 vertebra is noted (approximately at the level of the iliac crests). On either side of the spinous processes, this point is marked, and a second point 10 cm superior is also marked while the patient is still standing. The patient is then asked to bend forward, with knees extended. At the point of maximal flexion, the distance between the two points is re-measured. The difference between the first and second measurement is recorded.

IMAGING

If JAS is suspected, plain radiographs of the SI joints are required. Often a 30° tilt view is required to image the SI joint *en face*. Also AP and lateral views of the lumbosacral spine are helpful, which may include views in extremes of flexion and extension.

Early radiographic findings include changes of the SI joints (**59**). Later changes in the lumbar spine include 'squaring' and 'shiny corners,' which are radiographic findings that represent a proliferative process at areas of contact on the anterior longitudinal ligament and the anterior surface of the vertebral body (**60**).

These radiographic findings usually precede 'bamboo spine', which represents calcification of both the anterior and the posterior longitudinal spinal ligaments and is a very late finding (**61**).

Given that most JAS patients may not have axial symptoms, the frequency of radiographic changes at diagnosis of spine and SI joints is not clear. But even in those with axial symptoms who get conventional radiography, the frequency of characteristic changes of sacroiliitis of JAS is low. The ability of MRI to detect potential inflammatory changes around the SI joints early in the course of adults with AS that predict diagnostic radiographic changes years later has been recently demonstrated (Bennett *et al.* 2008). In this study, gradation of bone marrow edema adjacent to the SI joints was the best predictor of subsequent development of AS in a cohort of patients with IBP of less than 2 years' duration (better than B27 status) (Bennett *et al.* 2008). This important study may have significant implications for earlier diagnosis of JAS.

A study of nearly 80 patients with JAS and over 300 patients with AS with at least 20 years of disease duration confirmed earlier studies that axial radiographic changes are less in JAS compared with AS even with longer disease duration in the JAS cohort (Gensler *et al.* 2007).

DIFFERENTIAL DIAGNOSIS

Other conditions that present with inflammatory arthritis such as JRA/JIA share features with JAS, particularly if axial symptoms are absent. If enthesitis is present, other forms of JSpA should also be considered. Since peripheral inflammatory oligoarthritis ± enthesitis is a common presentation for JSpA in general and JAS in particular, specific questions about axial symptoms and assessment of spinal ROM are critical to avoid overlooking JAS in its early stages.

From an axial point of view, it is important to identify IBP from other forms of back pain. IBP is chronic as opposed to the acute back pain from injury or referred pain from urinary tract infection (UTI). Also IBP is better with activity as opposed to mechanical back pain, which is not. Back pain in a very young child, or that wakes the child from sleep is not likely to be from a spondyloarthropathy. Finally, there is stiffness in the back in the morning (or after prolonged rest, 'gelling') in IBP, which is not usually found in other forms of back pain.

PROGNOSIS

A cross-section of over 300 North American patients with JAS and 2000 patients with AS were assessed for functional status using the Bath Ankylosing Spondylitis Functional Index (BASFI) (Stone *et al.* 2005). In this study, those with JAS had longer duration of disease, greater delay in diagnosis, and higher BASFI scores (less function) than the AS cohort (Stone *et al.* 2005).

Also, JAS patients are at increased risk of developing severe hip involvement, as measured by an increased rate of total hip arthroplasty (Gensler *et al.* 2007). An example of the destructive hip arthropathy that can accompany JAS is shown (**62**).

MANAGEMENT

The important management principles for the axial features of JSpA, specifically JAS, are highlighted (**box 3**).

COMPLICATIONS

As with AS in adults, the primary potential complication of JAS is fusion of the spine and SI joints. The arthropathy in JAS is usually not destructive. Patients may also develop sequelae of uveitis, such as cataracts. In addition, complications of medical therapies such as gastritis associated with NSAIDs, infections associated with immunosuppressive medications, and bone disease related to corticosteroids may occur.

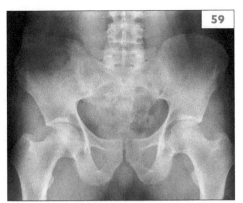

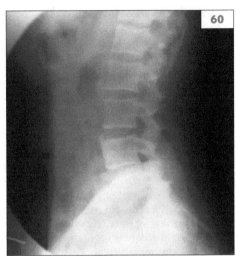

59–60 Unilateral sacroiliitis. In this AP view of the pelvis, the right SI joint has irregular margins, reactive sclerosis, primarily on the iliac side of the SI joint (**59**). 'Shiny corner.' In this lateral radiograph of the lumbar spine, the proliferative enthesitis, which has calcified, is apparent on the anterior edge of the L4 vertebral body. Earlier, more subtle changes of this process are also noted on the superior aspect of the anterior surface of the L2 vertebral body (**60**).

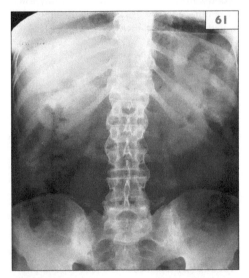

61–62 Unilateral sacroiliitis. 'Bamboo spine.' In this AP view of the lumbar spine, note the fusion of the SI joints, the preserved disc height, and the bilateral flowing calcifications ('dripping candle wax') from the proliferative enthesitis in this fused lumbar spine (**61**). Hip involvement. Severe right (R) hip disease that led to total hip arthroplasty within 1 year of this AP radiograph in this 34-year-old man with 10 years of AS. He was B27 positive, and although diagnosed at 24 years of age had had symptoms of AS from age 13 years (**62**).

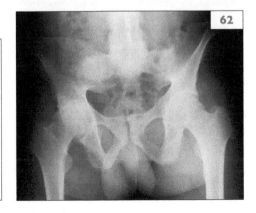

Box 3 Overview of the treatment of spine disease in JSpA

- Good posture
- Maintain ROM, encourage cervical extension
- Longitudinal assessments
- NSAIDs are treatment mainstay
- TNF blockers
- Intra-articular injections (SI)

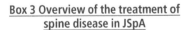

Juvenile psoriatic arthritis

DEFINITION
In 2004 a revised set of criteria were published for the diagnosis of JPsA (Petty *et al.* 2004), allowing a diagnosis of JPsA to be made if the child has psoriasis and arthritis or if the child has arthritis without psoriasis but fulfilled the criteria (*Table 9*).

EPIDEMIOLOGY AND ETIOLOGY
The overall prevalence of psoriasis is 1–3% and as many as one-third will develop it before age 16 years (Lewkowicz & Gottlieb 2004). The incidence of JPsA is about 3 cases per 100,000 children per year and has a prevalence of about 1/10,000 and accounts for up to 15% of children with chronic arthritis (Petty & Southwood 2005). The etiology of JPsA is unknown. It is not generally associated with HLA-B27 unless there is axial involvement (see below).

CLINICAL HISTORY
While most of the time psoriasis precedes the arthritis in adults, only 10–15% of children with JPsA have skin lesions at the time of diagnosis (Hafner & Michels 1996). The most common form of psoriasis in children is plaque psoriasis (Lewkowicz & Gottlieb 2004) (**63**). Another form is a predominantly guttate pattern of psoriasis, as shown in a 7-year-old boy at diagnosis (**64**).

Since the rash of psoriasis is frequently absent in children with JPsA, a careful inspection of the nails is important, as nail changes, particularly pitting (**65**, **66**), may precede the rash of psoriasis in these patients.

There seem to be two groups of children who get JPsA. One is younger, preschool-aged girls who generally have a polyarthritis and dactylitis; the other group is older boys who may have axial involvement or enthesitis and are more likely to have evidence of skin disease (Stoll & Nigrovic 2006).

PHYSICAL EXAMINATION
In those with peripheral arthritis, frequently joints involved will have a 'ray' distribution. This refers to joints in the same 'ray' of an extremity, such as the metacarpophalangeal (MCP), proximal interphalangeal (PIP), and distal interphalangeal (DIP) joints (**67**). When the joints are closer together, such as the toe, this is called dactylitis and may be referred to as a 'sausage digit', which is a characteristic feature of JPsA (**68**). Another feature of the arthritis of JPsA is the frequency of DIP involvement, more so than in other forms of arthritis. This is noted frequently in a DIP adjacent to a fingernail with active psoriatic changes.

LABORATORY
Routine laboratory studies such as CBC, ESR, and CRP may show evidence of an inflammatory process with elevations in the WBC, platelet count, ESR, and CRP along with evidence of the anemia of chronic disease. The presence of HLA-B27 increases the odds ratio for a diagnosis of a JSpA such as JPsA, particularly if there is axial involvement. As with the other forms of JSpA, autoantibodies are not frequently found in patients with JPsA; however, when they are found they are most likely to be low-titer ANA.

Table 9
Criteria for the diagnosis of juvenile psoriatic arthritis subgroup of juvenile idiopathic arthritis (Petty *et al.* 2004)

Diagnosis confirmed	Diagnosis confirmed	Exclusions
Arthritis *and* psoriasis	Arthritis *without* psoriasis, but with at least two of the following:	Family history in first-degree uveitis, AS, ReA, IBD-related sacroiliitis or enthesitis-related arthritis
	Dactylitis	Systemic-onset arthritis
	Nail changes	Positive RF
	Dermatologist confirmed psoriasis in at least one first-degree relative	B27 (+) boy older than 6 years

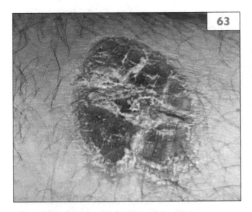

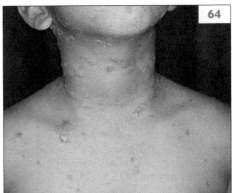

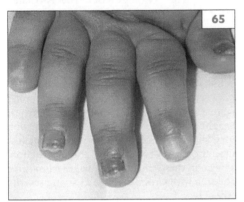

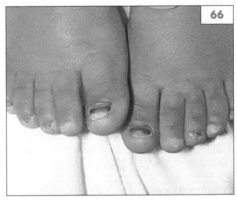

63–66 Psoriatic plaque. Oval-shaped, raised, scaly, hyperkeratotic lesion on the entensor surface of the leg of a young man with psoriasis (courtesy of Dawn M. R. Davis, MD, Mayo Clinic) (**63**); guttate distribution of psoriasis (courtesy of Dawn M. R. Davis, MD, Mayo Clinic) (**64**); nail pitting in a child with psoriasis. In the third and fourth fingernails, characteristic pitting is noted which may precede the development of arthritis (courtesy of Dawn M. R. Davis, MD, Mayo Clinic) (**65**); toenail changes in the child shown in **65**. Note the asymmetry (courtesy of Dawn M. R. Davis, MD, Mayo Clinic) (**66**).

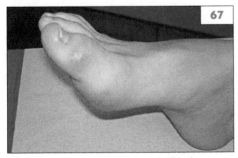

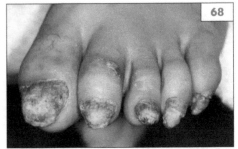

67 Inflammatory arthritis in right forefoot. Note the erythema and swelling over the medial aspects of the first metatarsophalangeal joint and interphalangeal joint of the great toe in this 14-year-old boy who was seronegative.

68 'Sausage' toe. Note the diffuse swelling of the second toe in this boy with severe nail changes from PsA (courtesy of C. J. Michet, MD, MPH, Mayo Clinic).

IMAGING

Since most patients with JPsA have peripheral joint involvement, they share imaging features with the other forms of JSpA.

DIFFERENTIAL DIAGNOSIS

With oligoarticular or axial presentation, the primary differential diagnosis is between the other forms of JSpA, enthesitis-related JIA and pauciarticular JRA (as discussed previously). The differential diagnosis of those with JPsA that present with polyarthritis includes polyarticular forms of JRA/JIA.

PROGNOSIS

Like most of the other forms of JSpA, the risk for erosive destructive arthritis in JPsA is low compared with JRA or JIA. As noted previously, however, the functional outcomes of children with JPsA seem to be worse than for children with other forms of chronic inflammatory arthritis (Selvaag *et al.* 2005).

MANAGEMENT

The principles of medical management of the peripheral musculoskeletal manifestations of JSpA such as JPsA are highlighted (**box 4**).

COMPLICATIONS

The arthropathy from JPsA is occasionally destructive. As with JAS, complications of medical therapies such as gastritis associated with NSAIDs, infections associated with immunosuppressive medications, and bone disease related to corticosteroids may occur.

Inflammatory bowel disease-associated arthropathy

DEFINITION

The peripheral or axial arthropathy associated with IBD such as ulcerative colitis or Crohn disease may be called IBD-associated arthropathy.

EPIDEMIOLOGY AND ETIOLOGY

Up to one-quarter of patients with IBD will have onset of disease before the age of 20 years (Burgos-Vargas *et al.* 1997). Joint disease, primarily arthralgias, has been reported in up to 20% of children with IBD (Lindsley & Laxer 2005). The etiology of IBD-associated arthropathy is unknown. It is not generally associated with HLA-B27 unless there is axial involvement.

CLINICAL HISTORY

While there are significant clinical differences between the common forms of IBD, similar features include abdominal pain, diarrhea, weight loss, and fever. Endoscopic examination may show a range of findings from shallow ulceration to 'cobblestoning' and obstruction, as seen in these endoscopic images from three children with Crohn disease of varying severity (**69–71**).

Box 4 Overview of the treatment of
peripheral arthritis in JSpA

- Maintain and improve ROM
- Longitudinal assessments
- NSAIDs are treatment mainstay
- Intra-articular injections
- DMARDS (sulfasalazine, methotrexate) as with JRA/JIA
- TNF blockers as with JRA/JIA

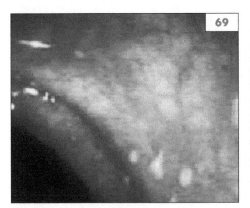

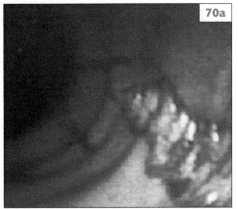

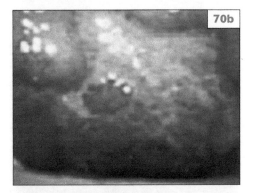

69–71 'Mild Crohn disease. Note the aphthous changes of the intestinal mucosa of the small intestine of this 14-year-old adolescent referred for intermittent loose stools and infrequent, mild abdominal pain (courtesy of W. A. Faubion, MD, Mayo Clinic) (**69**). Moderate Crohn disease. Note the erythematous borders and large areas of mucosal ulceration of the small bowel in this 12-year-old girl referred for diarrhea, abdominal pain, weight loss, and an abnormal small bowel radiograph (courtesy of W. A. Faubion, MD, Mayo Clinic) (**70a & b**). Severe Crohn disease. Cobblestoning and stricture formation is apparent in the small bowel of this 12-year-old girl referred for diarrhea, abdominal pain, growth retardation with anemia, and hypoalbuminemia (courtesy of W. A. Faubion, MD, Mayo Clinic) (**71**).

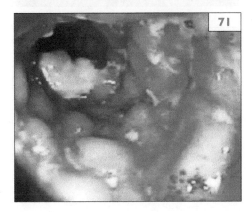

Painful skin lesions may be seen with IBD. One of these is erythema nodosa (EN). It is usually painful, subcutaneous, and frequently on the extensor surfaces of the legs (**72**). Another painful ulcerative lesion occasionally seen with IBD is pyoderma gangrenosum (**73**). Oral mucositis, which is painful, may precede the GI manifestations of IBD; a severe case of mucositis associated with Crohn disease is shown (**74**). Mucositis may be seen with other forms of JSpA.

PHYSICAL EXAMINATION

IBD-related arthropathy is primarily in the lower extremities (**75**), and is generally not as destructive as JRA (Burgos-Vargas *et al.* 1997). The axial disease seen in adults is very uncommon in children (Burgos-Vargas *et al.* 1997).

LABORATORY

Routine laboratory studies such as CBC, ESR, and CRP may show evidence of an inflamma-

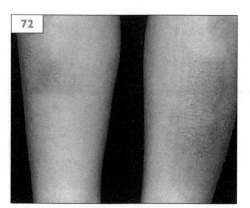

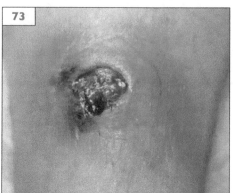

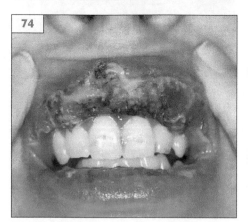

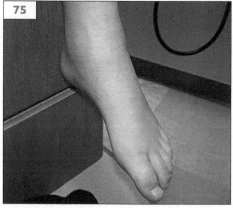

72–75 Erythema nodosa. These slightly raised, painful subcutaneous lesions may be seen in patients with IBD (courtesy of Dawn M. R. Davis, MD, Mayo Clinic) (**72**). Pyoderma gangrenosum. This ulcerating lesion, usually on the lower extremities may be seen in patients with IBD (courtesy of Dawn M. R. Davis, MD, Mayo Clinic) (**73**). Mucositis in Crohn disease. Very severe oral mucositis in a woman with Crohn disease of 7 years' duration (courtesy of W. A. Faubion, MD, Mayo Clinic) (**74**). Large left ankle effusion. Synovial overgrowth and synovial fluid are palpable and warm in this 8-year-old boy with seronegative oligoarthritis, who had an antalgic gait (**75**).

tory process with elevations in the WBC, platelet count, ESR, and CRP along with evidence of the anemia of chronic disease. Evidence of occult blood is frequently found in stool samples. Autoantibodies are uncommon.

IMAGING
Although clinical features and endoscopic evaluations are the mainstay of diagnosing IBD, imaging can assist the diagnostic process. In addition to excluding other reasons for the symptoms of enteritis, abdominal imaging such as CT scanning can show inflammatory findings such as bowel wall thickening (**76a, b**).

Since most patients with IBD-associated arthropathy have peripheral joint involvement, they share imaging features with the other forms of JSpA.

DIFFERENTIAL DIAGNOSIS
Since IBD-associated arthropathy occurs with or after the diagnosis of IBD, the primary differential diagnosis of a peripheral arthritis would include infectious (septic) arthritis or post-infectious (reactive) arthritis. The differential diagnosis of axial IBD-associated arthropathy would include the other forms of JSpA.

PROGNOSIS
Like most of the other forms of JSpA, the risk for erosive, destructive arthritis in IBD-associated arthropathy is low compared with JRA or JIA. Few data are available on the long-term functional outcomes of children with IBD-associated arthropathy.

MANAGEMENT
The principles of medical management of the peripheral musculoskeletal manifestations of JPsA such as the arthropathy associated with IBD are highlighted (see **box 4**). One of the challenges of managing these patients is that many are not candidates for NSAIDs because of their potential for adverse actions to the GI system.

COMPLICATIONS
The arthropathy in IBD-associated arthropathy is usually not destructive. Patients may rarely develop sequelae of uveitis, such as cataracts. Complications of medical therapies such as infections associated with immunosuppressive

medications may occur. Bone disease related to corticosteroids may be enhanced by vitamin and mineral deficiencies related to enteritis. Poorly controlled IBD can increase the risk of bowel perforation, fistulae formation, and growth retardation.

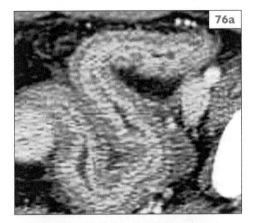

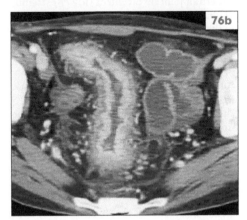

76a, b Severe Crohn disease. Selected images from CT scan of the small bowel of the 12-year-old girl (see **70a & b**) show the marked bowel wall thicking and inflammation evident on endoscopy (courtesy of W. A. Faubion, MD, Mayo Clinic).

REACTIVE ARTHROPATHIES

The hallmarks of reactive arthropathies are its post-infectious nature and its absence of infection in the joints affected (**box 5**).

Reactive arthritis

DEFINITION
ReA is a sterile inflammatory arthritis that occurs after an identifiable non-streptococcal infectious exposure.

EPIDEMIOLOGY AND ETIOLOGY
Estimates of the relative frequency of ReA in several pediatric rheumatology series ranges from around 10% to 40%, based on the criteria used (Burgos-Varga & Vazquez-Mellado 2005). The precise mechanisms of how the infectious agents in ReA initiate a remote, inflammatory response are not known, but depend on both host and pathogen characteristics.

CLINICAL HISTORY
ReA usually follows a pathogenic enteric bacterial infection or a lower UTI with *Chlamydia*. Post-enteric ReA tends to occur in younger children and the post-UTI form is seen more in adolescents and young adults. The pattern of joint involvement (lower extremity, oligoarthritis, asymmetric, and so on) is similar to the other forms of JSpA. Enthesitis may also be present. The involved joints are very painful.

PHYSICAL EXAMINATION
An oligoarthritis with acutely swollen, tender lower extremity joints (see **75**) would be characteristic of ReA. Lower extremity enthesitis or dactylitis may also be seen. Findings of inflammatory eye disease, such as uveitis, may also be seen. The classic form of ReA is characterized by urethritis, conjunctivitis, and a painful oligoarthritis frequently following a lower UTI.

Two characteristic skin findings may be seen in older children with ReA. In males, circinate balanitis may be seen in a few cases of ReA (**77**). Keratoderma blenorrhagicum is a pustlar rash, on the soles of feet and may also be seen in an occasional patient with ReA (**78**).

LABORATORY
Routine laboratory studies such as CBC, ESR, and CRP may show evidence of an inflammatory process with elevations in the WBC, platelet count, ESR, and CRP along with evidence of the anemia of chronic disease. The presence of HLA-B27 increases the odds ratio of a diagnosis of ReA, particularly if there is axial involvement.

Since the time between the exposure and the development of arthritis could be several weeks, or the exposure may have generated minimal symptoms, a very high degree of suspicion is needed to look for potential GI or GU pathogens that could be provocative. Stool culture and urine polymerase chain reaction for evidence of previous chlamydia infection may be needed.

IMAGING
Since most patients with ReA have peripheral joint involvement, they share imaging features with the other forms of JSpA.

DIFFERENTIAL DIAGNOSIS
The primary concern is to be sure that the child has a post-infectious ReA and not an infectious form of arthritis, such as septic arthritis. Additionally the arthropathy of ReA shares many features of the other forms of JSpA.

PROGNOSIS
Like most of the other forms of JspA, the risk for erosive destructive arthritis in ReA is low compared with JRA or JIA. Few data are available on the functional outcomes of children with ReA.

MANAGEMENT
The management principles and frequently used medications for ReA are shown (**box 6**). The use of antibiotics (beyond treating the initial, precipitating infection) to treat the arthritis of ReA is not felt to be helpful (Kvien *et al.* 2004).

COMPLICATIONS
The arthropathy in ReA is usually not destructive. Patients may also develop sequelae of uveitis, such as cataracts. Like JPsA, complications of medical therapies such as gastritis associated with NSAIDs, infections associated with immunosuppressive medications, and bone disease related to corticosteroids may occur.

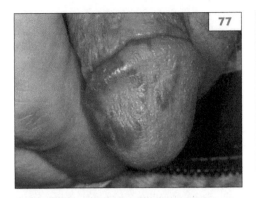

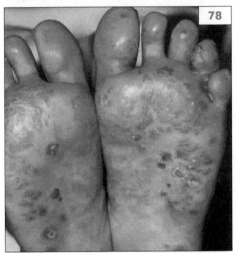

77, 78 Circinate balanitis. This rash, which is usually painless, may be seen in a subset of males with ReA (courtesy of Dawn M. R. Davis, MD, Mayo Clinic) (**77**). Keratoderma blenorrhagicum. This painless, pustular rash on the soles of the feet may be seen in Reiter syndrome, a form of ReA (courtesy of Dawn M. R. Davis, MD, Mayo Clinic) (**78**).

Box 5 Keys to recognizing juvenile reactive arthropathies including ReA, ARF, and PSRA

- Acute, very painful, sterile arthritis
- After an identifiable exposure
- Typical exposures include enteropathic bacteria and *Chlamydia*
- Post-streptococcal conditions like rheumatic fever and PSRA are also reactive arthropathies

---

Box 6 Overview of the treatment of ReA

- Identify the exposure, treat as indicated
- Exclude septic arthritis
- NSAIDs are the treatment mainstay
- Longitudinal assessments
- Intra-articular injections
- DMARDs (sulfasalazine, methotrexate) rarely

POST-STREPTOCOCCAL ARTHROPATHIES

Acute rheumatic fever

DEFINITION
Acute rheumatic fever (ARF) is defined by the Jones criteria established in 1944 (Jones 1944), which are characterized by major and minor criteria (*Table 10*) (Dajani *et al.* 1992).

EPIDEMIOLOGY AND ETIOLOGY
Although estimates of the incidence of ARF in developing countries may be as high as 100 cases per 100,000 per year, the incidence rate in the US is 0.5–3 cases per 100,000 children per year (Ayoub & Alsaeid 2005). The precise mechanisms of how the infectious agents in ARF initiate a remote, inflammatory response are not known, but depend on both host and pathogen characteristics.

CLINICAL HISTORY
ARF follows a group A ß-hemolytic streptococcal (GABHS) upper respiratory infection (URI). This form of reactive arthropathy tends to have a migratory pattern, with primarily large joint involvement. In both ARF and ReA, the joint pain is generally out of proportion to physical findings.

PHYSICAL EXAMINATION
In adults the joint disease may be the primary clinical feature; in children cardiac involvement is more common. Insufficiency murmurs may be noted. The rash of erythema marginatum (79) is uncommon as are subcutaneous nodules. A late finding of rheumatic fever is chorea, which is also very uncommon. It may present months after the initial GABHS URI, and be a challenge to link to ARF.

LABORATORY
Routine laboratory studies such as CBC, ESR, and CRP may show evidence of an inflammatory process with elevations in the WBC, platelet count, ESR, and CRP and evidence of the anemia of chronic disease.

Documenting the recent URI with GABHS can be done with microbiologic techniques such as 'rapid-strep' screens or throat cultures. Alternatively, serologic studies may be preferred. Elevated serum titers of anti-streptococcal antibodies such as ASO or DNase B document a recent GABHS exposure. Unlike JSpA and ReA, there is no association with HLA-B27.

An ECG is done to document cardiac conduction abnormalities or other markers of structural cardiac damage.

IMAGING
Like the other forms of reactive arthropathies, the risk of joint damage is very low, and imaging affected joints may show evidence of soft tissue swelling, but no joint space narrowing or erosion.

Imaging of the heart with echocardiography is very important in assessing potential cardiac disease in ARF. While myocardial and pericardial disease may be present, the primary purpose of echocardiography is to assess for potential valvular abnormalities.

Table 10
Modified Jones criteria for the diagnosis of acute rheumatic fever (Dajani *et al.* 1992)

The diagnosis of ARF is made when at least two major or two minor and one major criteria are present following a group A, β-hemolytic streptococcal URI.

Major criteria	Minor criteria	Previous strep URI
Carditis	Fever	Increased Strep Ab titers
Arthritis	Arthralgia culture	(+) throat
Sydenham chorea	Increased ESR	(+) rapid strep screen
Erythema marginatum	Increased CRP	
Subcutaneous skin nodules	Prolonged PR interval	

Strep Ab, antistreptococcal antibodies such as ASO and anti-deoxynuclease B (DNase B).

DIFFERENTIAL DIAGNOSIS

The primary diagnosis in the differential is post-streptococcal reactive arthritis (PSRA) if the arthropathy is post-streptococcal. Higher levels of acute-phase reactants and more treatment-resistant arthropathy favor the diagnosis of ARF (Barash *et al.* 2008). Also, the arthropathy of PSRA is not migratory like ARF. Other forms of ReA may have similar clinical features.

PROGNOSIS

Like most of the other forms of reactive arthropathies, the risk for erosive destructive arthritis in ARF is extremely low compared with JRA or JIA. The presence of valvular heart disease is the primary prognostic marker. Because the valvular disease can progress with repeated GABHS exposures, antibiotic prophylaxis is indicated (see below).

MANAGEMENT

Penicillin is the primary treatment for the acute URI and skin infections with GABHS responsible for ARF and PSRA. The American Heart Association (AHA) has guidelines for antibiotic prophylaxis for the prevention of progression of valvular heart disease in patients with rheumatic fever (Dajani *et al.* 1995).

The management of the arthropathy of post-streptococcal arthropathies, including ARF, is highlighted (**box 7**).

COMPLICATIONS

The arthropathy in ARF is not destructive. Complications of NSAID use include gastritis and renal insufficiency. The primary potential extra-articular complication is valvular heart disease.

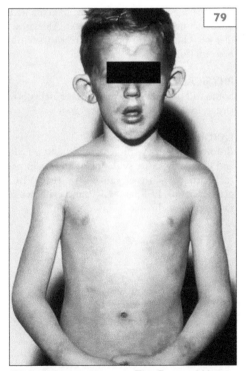

79 Erythema marginatum. This 7-year-old boy had a widespread rash, including involvement of his face, following a recent streptococcal URI (courtesy of Lisa Drage, MD, Mayo Clinic).

Box 7 Overview of the treatment of ARF and PSRA

- Identify GABHS URI and treat if indicated
- Assess for extra-articular involvement
- NSAIDs are the treatment mainstay
- Extensive antibiotic prophylaxis if ARF, some antibiotic prophylaxis if PSRA

Post-streptococcal reactive arthritis

DEFINITION

Post-streptococcal reactive arthritis is a reactive arthropathy that follows a streptococcal URI, but doesn't meet the criteria for ARF. Criteria for the diagnosis for PSRA (Ayoub & Ahmed 1997) are shown (*Table 11*).

EPIDEMIOLOGY AND ETIOLOGY

The incidence of PSRA may be 1–2 cases per 100,000 children per year, and was about twice as frequent as ARF in a US study (Ayoub & Alsaeid 2005). The precise mechanisms of how the infectious agents in PSRA initiate a remote, inflammatory response are not known, but are similar to ARF.

CLINICAL HISTORY

While similar to ARF as a post-streptococcal reactive arthropathy, PSRA differs from ARF in that the joint involvement is not migratory, and is more persistent in PSRA. Since patients with PSRA cannot have other features of ARF, heart disease, chorea, and nodules are not seen at presentation.

PHYSICAL EXAMINATION

Some will have fever and most have arthritis in larger, lower extremity joints.

LABORATORY

Routine laboratory studies such as CBC, ESR, and CRP may show evidence of an inflammatory process with elevations in the WBC, platelet count, ESR, and CRP, and evidence of the anemia of chronic disease.

Documenting the recent URI with GABHS can be done with microbiologic techniques such as 'rapid-strep' screens or throat cultures. Alternatively, serologic studies may be preferred. Elevated serum titers of anti-streptococcal antibodies such as ASO or DNase B document a recent GABHS exposure. Unlike JSpA and ReA, there is no association with HLA-B27.

IMAGING

Like the other forms of reactive arthropathies, the risk of joint damage is very low, and imaging affected joints may show evidence of soft tissue swelling, but no joint space narrowing or erosion.

DIFFERENTIAL DIAGNOSIS

The primary diagnosis in the differential is rheumatic fever if the arthropathy is post-streptococcal. As noted previously, higher levels of acute phase reactants and more treatment-resistant arthropathy favor the diagnosis of ARF (Barash *et al.* 2008). Since the arthropathy of PSRA is not migratory like ARF, it could be confused with polyarticular forms of JRA/JIA.

PROGNOSIS

Like rheumatic fever, the risk for erosive destructive arthritis in PSRA is extremely low compared with JRA or JIA. Cases of carditis have been described following the diagnosis of PSRA, thus antibiotic prophylaxis is indicated (see below).

MANAGEMENT

Penicillin is also the primary treatment for the acute URI with GABHS responsible for PSRA.

The duration of antibiotic prophylaxis in patients who have had PSRA is unclear, but one reference suggests prophylaxis for 1 year after diagnosis (Dajani *et al.* 1995).

The management of the arthropathy of post-streptococcal arthropathies, including PSRA, is highlighted (**box 7**).

COMPLICATIONS

The arthropathy in PSRA is not destructive. Complications of NSAID use include gastritis and renal insufficiency. PSRA is not associated with cardiac involvement.

Table 11
Proposed criteria for the diagnosis of post-streptococcal reactive arthritis (Ayoub & Ahmed 1997)

The diagnosis of PSRA may be made when an arthritis following a group A ß-hemolytic streptococcal (GABHS) URI occurs with these features and doesn't meet the criteria for acute rheumatic fever (ARF).

Characteristics of arthritis	Evidence of GABHS URI	Exclusions
Acute-onset, non-migratory	Rapid strep screen	Any major criteria for ARF
Persistent or recurrent	Throat culture	Meets criteria for ARF
Suboptimal response to aspirin or NSAIDs	Strep Ab	

Strep Ab, antistreptococcal antibodies such as ASO and antideoxynuclease B (DNase B).

CHAPTER 4

Lupus erythematosus

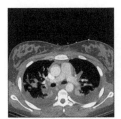 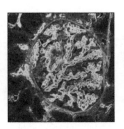 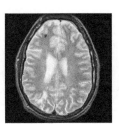 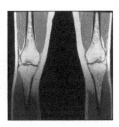

Systemic lupus erythematosus

DEFINITION

Systemic lupus erythematosus (SLE) is a heterogeneous, inflammatory, autoimmune disorder affecting multiple organ systems, which causes significant morbidity and mortality. Although its etiology, pathogenesis, clinical findings, and laboratory abnormalities are similar to adult-onset SLE, children affected with lupus have special considerations regarding physical and emotional growth and development, treatment toxicities, and lifelong burden of chronic disease. Childhood-onset SLE (onset <16 years of age) makes up approximately 15–20% of all SLE cases, and pediatric lupus is more severe than adult-onset SLE, having a more aggressive presentation and course, including more frequent renal involvement (Barron *et al.* 1993, Carreno *et al.* 1999, Tucker *et al.* 1995).

EPIDEMIOLOGY AND ETIOLOGY

The incidence and prevalence of SLE vary with geographic location and race/ethnicity. The estimated incidence of pediatric SLE is 0.6 per 100,000 (Fessel 1988). Lupus occurs throughout the world, and may be more frequent in non-white populations. For example, Asians, African–Americans, and Hispanics have a higher incidence of SLE compared with whites (Rus & Hochberg 2002). These racial/ethnic groups may also have a more severe disease course. SLE, like many autoimmune diseases, is more common in females than males.

The etiology of SLE is complex and incompletely understood. In a genetically susceptible individual, there is loss of normal homeostatic control of immunologic reactivity to antigens.

SLE is an autoimmune disease characterized by production of antibodies against the patient's own nuclear and cellular components. The triggers for the formation of these antibodies are still under investigation, but may include environmental factors, such as infections, UV light, and drug exposure. There may be decreased clearance of apoptotic cellular debris, causing self-antigens to be abnormally presented, triggering autoantibody formation and immune complex deposition (**80**). The immune complexes may be ineffectively cleared, resulting in cytokine release, inappropriate inflammation, and tissue destruction (**81**). Hormonal factors are also implicated, given the female-to-male predominance.

There is some evidence for a genetic susceptibility, with increased concordance of SLE among identical twins (Deapen *et al.* 1992). In approximately 10% of families with a lupus diagnosis, another connective tissue disease can be found. This illustrates the heritability of lupus, but the actual susceptibility to SLE is multifactorial and polygenic. Lupus predisposition is associated with selective IgA deficiency, the C4A null allele, and inherited complement deficiencies, such as C2, C1q, C1r, and C1 esterase inhibitor. HLA-DR3 and HLA-DR2 increase the risk of SLE in whites, and HLA-DR2 is associated in African–Americans with SLE (Cassidy & Petty 2005).

Drugs thought to classically induce a lupus-like syndrome include hydralazine, minocycline, and some anticonvulsants. However, many drugs have been implicated with this phenomenon. Often, the clinical symptoms of drug-induced lupus will resolve with discontinuation of the offending trigger. Drug-induced lupus is associated with anti-histone antibodies.

80 Pathogenesis of SLE.

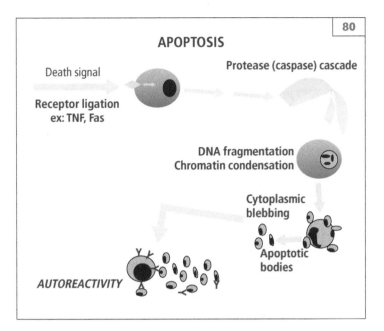

81 Pathogenesis of SLE.
RBC, red blood cell; BM, basement membrane.

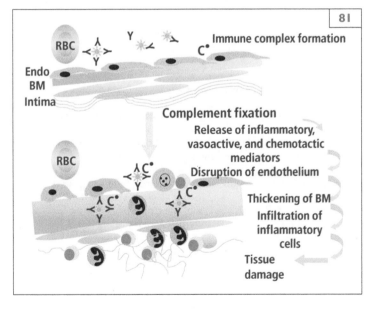

CLINICAL HISTORY

The American College of Rheumatology (ACR) revised diagnostic criteria for SLE in 1982 and again in 1997 (*Table 12*) (Hochberg 1997, Tan *et al.* 1982, Weening *et al.* 2004). In adults, SLE is diagnosed when 4 of the 11 criteria are met. The 1982 criteria have been validated in children with a sensitivity and specificity of 96% (Cassidy & Petty 2005). Patients who do not meet the full diagnostic criteria for SLE are often followed in a pediatric rheumatology clinic because as many as 50% of them will eventually meet the diagnostic criteria (Hallengran *et al.* 2004).

Constitutional symptoms such as fevers, malaise, and weight loss are common at disease presentation and with flares of disease activity. Musculoskeletal involvement may include arthralgias or arthritis that is usually non-erosive and non-deforming. Osteoporosis and avascular necrosis (**82, 83**) can also be seen and may be a complication of treatment with chronic corticosteroids. Raynaud phenomenon is a common vascular manifestation and is characterized by vasospasm of the extremities leading to red, white, and/or blue color changes, often triggered by cold or stress.

Table 12
American College of Rheumatology classification criteria for diagnosis of systemic lupus erythematosus

The 1997 Revised Criteria for Classification of SLE*

Criterion	Definition
1. Malar rash	Fixed erythema, flat or raised, over the malar eminences, tending to spare the nasolabial folds
2. Discoid rash	Erythematous raised patches with adherent keratotic scaling and follicular plugging; atrophic scarring may occur in older lesions
3. Photosensitivity	Skin rash as a result of unusual reaction to sunlight, by patient history or physician observation
4. Oral ulcers	Oral or nasopharyngeal ulceration, usually painless, observed by physician
5. Arthritis	Non-erosive arthritis involving two or more peripheral joints, characterized by tenderness, swelling, or effusion
6. Serositis	(a) Pleuritis – convincing history of pleuritic pain or rubbing heard by a physician or evidence of pleural effusion OR (b) Pericarditis – documented by ECG or rub or evidence of pericardial effusion
7. Renal disorder	(a) Persistent proteinuria greater than 0.5 grams per day or greater than 3+ if quantitation not performed OR (b) Cellular casts – may be red cell, hemoglobin, granular, tubular, or mixed
8. Neurologic disorder	(a) Seizures – in the absence of offending drugs or known metabolic derangements, e.g. uremia, ketoacidosis, or electrolyte imbalance OR (b) Psychosis – in the absence of offending drugs or known metabolic derangements, e.g. uremia, ketoacidosis, or electrolyte imbalance

9. Hematologic disorder	(a) Hemolytic anemia – with reticulocytosis OR (b) Leukopenia – less than 4,000/mm^3 total on two or more occasions OR (c) Lymphopenia – less than 1,500/mm^3 on two or more occasions OR (d) Thrombocytopenia – less than 100,000/mm^3 in the absence of offending drugs
10. Immunologic disorder	(a) Anti-DNA – antibody to native DNA in abnormal titer OR (b) Anti-Sm – presence of antibody to Sm nuclear antigen OR (c) Positive finding of antiphospholipid antibodies based on: (1) an abnormal serum level of IgG or IgM anticardiolipin antibodies (2) a positive test result for lupus anticoagulant using a standard method, or (3) a false-positive serologic test for syphilis known to be positive for at least 6 months and confirmed by *Treponema pallidum* immobilization or fluorescent treponemal antibody absorption test
11. ANA	An abnormal titer of ANA by immunofluorescence or an equivalent assay at any point in time and in the absence of drugs known to be associated with 'drug-induced lupus' syndrome

* The proposed classification is based on 11 criteria. For the purpose of identifying patients in clinical studies, a person shall be said to have SLE if any 4 or more of the 11 criteria are present, serially or simultaneously, during any interval of observation.

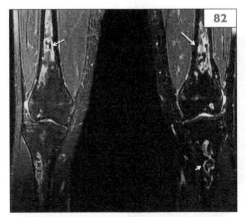

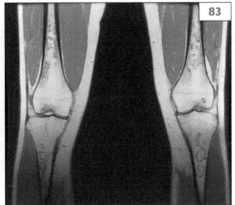

82 MRI T2-weighted image with fat saturation of an adolescent with SLE after high-dose pulse steroid administration with subsequent avascular necrosis of her femurs and tibias (courtesy of Ann M. Reed, MD, Mayo Clinic).

83 MRI T1-weighted image of an adolescent with SLE after high-dose pulse steroid administration with subsequent avascular necrosis of her femurs and tibias (courtesy of Ann M. Reed, MD, Mayo Clinic).

Cardiac abnormalities in patients with lupus range from pericarditis (**84, 85**) and myocarditis to Libman–Sacks endocarditis and coronary artery disease. Pericarditis may manifest as recurrent chest pain and shortness of breath. Lupus is an additional independent risk factor for atherosclerosis, and adult lupus patients can have myocardial infarctions earlier than the general population (Deapen *et al.* 1992, Manzi *et al.* 1997).

The most common pulmonary lesions in SLE are pleural effusions which may present with pleuritic chest pain or shortness of breath (**86**). Pulmonary function testing is followed and lupus patients most commonly develop a restrictive pattern. When pulmonary hemorrhage occurs, it can be life threatening. Pulmonary emboli from antibodies against cardiolipin or a lupus anticoagulant can also cause shortness of breath and chest pain (**87, 88**).

Liver dysfunction in the form of acute autoimmune hepatitis is the most frequent liver pathology related to SLE; however, steatohepatitis is common secondary to steroid use and obesity (**89**).

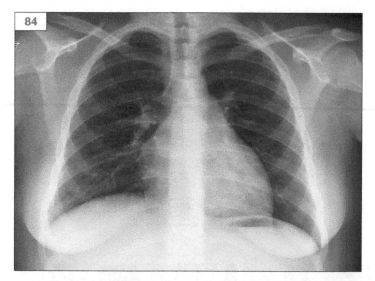

84 Pericardial effusion presenting with shortness of breath and anterior chest pain which needed drainage and pericardial tube (courtesy of Ann M. Reed, MD, Mayo Clinic).

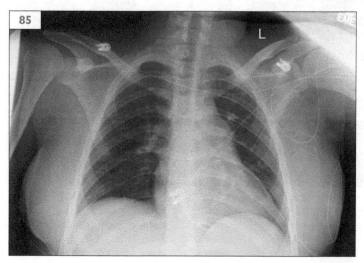

85 Pericardial effusion after pericardial drain.

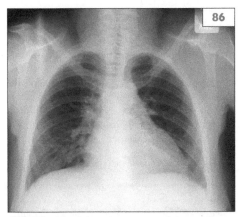

86 SLE with slight enlargement of the cardiac silhouette felt to be related to a pleural effusion.

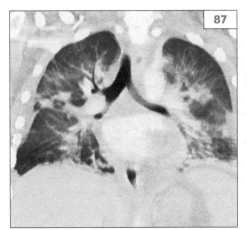

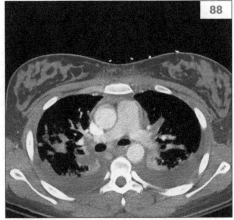

87–89 Diffuse pulmonary emboli in a patient with anticardiolipin antibody (87); CT scan demonstrating pulmonary artery thrombosis (88); CT scan of the liver showing diffuse fatty infiltrate in a patient with lupus on high-dose steroids (89).

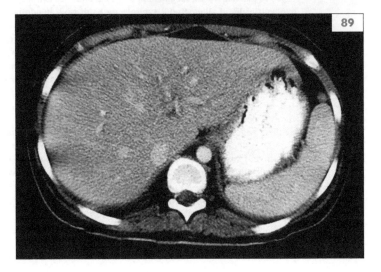

Renal involvement is a common complication in both adults and children, although it is more prevalent in pediatric-onset SLE. When present, nephritis in children is often more severe than in adults with SLE. It can show at presentation or develop many years later. Patients with nephritis present with hematuria and proteinuria. Hypertension or edema may be present. Children commonly have a renal biopsy to evaluate the extent of lupus involvement if they present with or develop abnormalities in their urinalysis. Lupus nephritis has been most recently reclassified in 2003 by the International Society of Nephrology/Renal Pathology Society (ISN/RPS) into classes I–VI (*Table 13*) (Weening *et al.* 2004). Of these, class IV lupus nephritis, which is diffuse, proliferative glomerulonephritis, is the most common and severe (**90–94**) (Emre *et al.* 2001).

Table 13
International Society Nephrology/Renal Pathology Society 2003 Classification of Lupus Nephritis (adapted from Weening *et al.* 2004)

Indicate and grade (mild, moderate, severe) tubular atrophy, interstitial inflammation, and fibrosis, severity of arteriosclerosis, or other vascular lesions.

Class I	Minimal mesangial lupus nephritis Normal glomeruli by light microscopy, but mesangial immune deposits by immunofluorescence
Class II	Mesangial proliferative lupus nephritis Purely mesangial hypercellularity of any degree or mesangial matrix expansion by light microscopy, with mesangial immune deposits. There may be a few isolated subepithelial or subendothelial deposits visible by immunofluorescence or electron microscopy, but not by light microscopy
Class III	Focal lupus nephritis Active or inactive focal, segmental or global endo- or extracapillary glomerulonephritis involving <50% of all glomeruli, typically with focal subendothelial immune deposits, with or without mesangial alterations. A, active lesions; A/C, active and chronic lesions; C, chronic lesions
Class IV	Diffuse lupus nephritis Active or inactive diffuse, segmental, or global endo- or extracapillary glomerulonephritis involving ≥50% of all glomeruli, typically with diffuse subendothelial immune deposits, with or without mesangial alterations. This class is divided into diffuse segmental (IV-S) lupus nephritis when ≥50% of the involved glomeruli have segmental lesions, and diffuse global (IV-G) lupus nephritis when ≥50% of the involved glomeruli have global lesions. Segmental is defined as a glomerular lesion that involves less than half of the glomerular tuft. This class includes cases with diffuse wire loop deposits but with little or no glomerular proliferation. A, active lesions; A/C, active and chronic lesions; C, chronic lesions
Class V	Membranous lupus nephritis Global or segmental subepithelial immune deposits or their morphologic sequelae by light microscopy and immunofluorescence or electron microscopy, with or without mesangial alterations. Class V lupus nephritis may occur in combination with class III or IV in which case both will be diagnosed. Class V lupus nephritis may show advanced sclerosis
Class VI	Advanced sclerosing lupus nephritis ≥90% of glomeruli globally sclerosed without residual activity

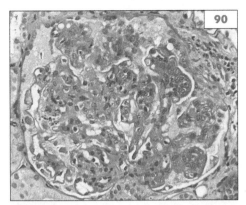

90 Class IV lupus glomerulonephritis (light microscopy).

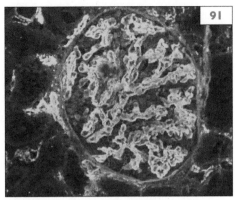

91 Class IV lupus glomerulonephritis (immunofluorescence) (courtesy of Sanjeev Sethi, MD, PhD, Mayo Clinic).

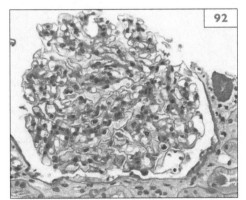

92 Class II mild mesangial proliferative lupus glomerulonephritis (courtesy of Sanjeev Sethi, MD, PhD, Mayo Clinic).

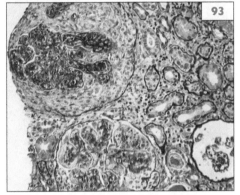

93 Lupus crescentic glomerulonephritis (courtesy of Sanjeev Sethi, MD, PhD, Mayo Clinic).

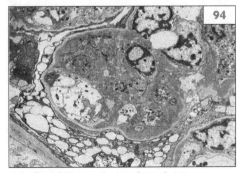

94 Class IV lupus glomerulonephritis subendothelial deposits (electron microscopy) (courtesy of Sanjeev Sethi, MD, PhD, Mayo Clinic).

Lupus involvement of the central nervous system (CNS) is sometimes difficult to diagnose and the symptoms are very non-specific. Symptoms such as poor concentration, poor school performance, memory loss, depression, headache, and visual or auditory hallucinations should be evaluated in a patient with SLE. More serious symptoms can include seizures, strokes, bleeds, or coma (**95–99**). Neuropsychiatric testing can be helpful to make the diagnosis and to follow progress. Evaluation, especially for school, must be tailored to the child's age and

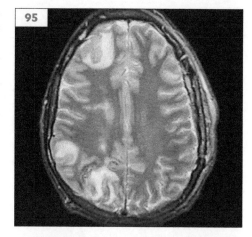

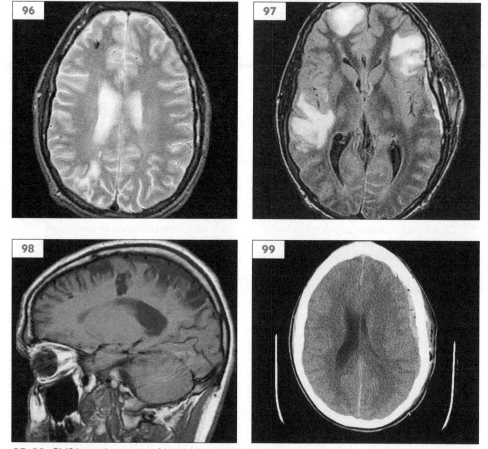

95–99 CNS lupus (courtesy of Ann M. Reed, MD, Mayo Clinic) (**95**); stroke in a teenager with CNS lupus (**96**); CNS infarcts with lupus patient and antifactor antibodies to factor 2 (**97**); CNS infarcts: a child with new-onset SLE and antifactor antibodies (**98**); subdural bleed in an SLE patient with a midline shift (**99**).

developmental level. Patients with a chronic disease, such as SLE, are at high risk for depression, which can sometimes be difficult to distinguish from neuropsychiatric lupus.

PHYSICAL EXAMINATION

Cutaneous manifestations include malar (butterfly) rash, discoid rash, periungal erythema, mucosal ulcerations, photosensitivity, cutaneous erythema (**100**), and alopecia. The malar rash (**101, 101b**) is the most common cutaneous manifestation and is present over the nasal bridge, extends onto the cheeks, and spares the nasolabial folds. It is often symmetric and well demarcated, slightly raised, and with texture. Petechiae (**102**) and purpura (**103**) can be related to vasculitis or underlying thrombocytopenia.

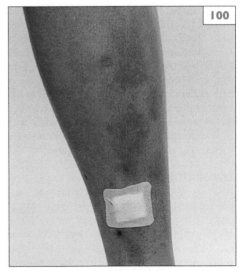

100 Cutaneous erythema in a patient with new-onset lupus (courtesy of Ann M. Reed, MD, Mayo Clinic).

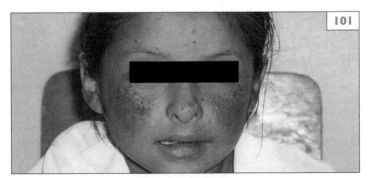
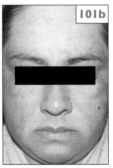

101, 101b Malar rash (courtesy of Ann M. Reed, MD, Mayo Clinic) (**101**); malar rash (**101b**).

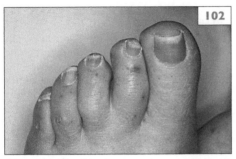
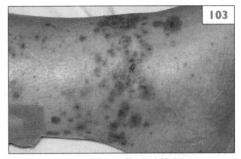

102, 103 Petechiae from a patient with SLE and vasculitis (courtesy of Dawn Davis, MD, Mayo Clinic) (**102**); purpura in a child with SLE and vasculitis (courtesy of Dawn Davis, MD, Mayo Clinic) (**103**).

The classic mucosal involvement of patients with SLE is a shallow, painless ulceration (**104**) of the hard palate with surrounding erythema. Ulcerations present in the oral or nasal mucosa can be painful, especially when present on the tongue. These ulcerations are not as specific for SLE. Edema may be a sign of renal involvement. Joint swelling, tenderness, and limited ROM are indicators of arthritis in children with SLE. Serositis may be detected on exam by the presence of pleural or pericardial rubs.

LABORATORY

ANA is the most common autoantibody present in SLE patients and is present in 98% of children with SLE (Worrall *et al.* 1990). ANAs are present in 10–15% of healthy children and can be increased non-specifically with infections, but usually to a low titer. More specific ANAs common in SLE include anti-dsDNA, anti-SSA (anti-Ro), anti-SSB (anti-La), anti-Smith, and anti-histone antibodies. Only the ANA, dsDNA, and Smith antibodies are part of the ACR diagnostic criteria. The dsDNA antibodies can be followed over time, because they correlate with increased active systemic inflammation and lupus nephritis in particular. Ribonuclear protein (RNP) antibodies can be present in patients with SLE in low titers and with mixed connective tissue disease (MCTD) in high titers.

Hematologic abnormalities are frequently seen in SLE patients at presentation and with flares of disease. Anemia in SLE patients can be either hemolytic or anemia of chronic disease. A Coombs test will likely be positive in patients with hemolytic anemia due to IgG complement fixing antibodies against red blood cells (Cassidy & Petty 2005). Pancytopenia can also be present. Patients who develop thrombotic thrombocytopenic purpura require hospitalization and aggressive treatment because this can be fatal.

Coagulation abnormalities in SLE patients can be due to either the presence of anti-phospholipid (APL) antibodies, such as a lupus anticoagulant, or anti-cardiolipin antibodies. APL antibodies and the lupus anticoagulant are measured in a number of ways and must be present on at least two occasions 12 weeks apart for the ACR diagnostic criteria. SLE patients can have thrombosis and bleeding at the same time, making them difficult to treat.

SLE patients with active systemic inflammation often have increased non-specific markers of inflammation such as an elevated ESR. C3 and C4 complements are consumed by the circulating immune complexes and are often low in SLE patients with active disease. C3 and C4 are followed clinically, because decreases in these components of the complement cascade correlate with systemic disease activity.

Urinalysis is done regularly with a random urine protein-to-creatinine ratio to monitor for development of nephritis. Active renal disease is indicated by an increase in the first morning urine protein:creatinine ratio, hematuria, pyuria, or the presence of urinary casts. Renal biopsies are commonly done in children with SLE to characterize the ISN/RPS classification, activity and chronicity of renal involvement (*Table 14*), which helps guide treatment options.

IMAGING

There is no specific imaging test pathognomonic for lupus; instead, radiological studies can only support or challenge the suspicion of this diagnosis. For example, chest radiographs may show pleural effusion or an enlarged heart consistent with pericardial effusions characteristic of the serositis seen in lupus. Joint radiographs and MR images may show soft-tissue swelling and joint fluid, but the arthritis of lupus is usually nonerosive and easily treated. A kidney ultrasound may be required if there is nephritis, or an abdominal ultrasound if there are liver function test abnormalities. A head MR scan and/or MR angiogram is recommended for concerns of lupus cerebritis. For treatment-related toxicities, bone density scans help to evaluate the bone health of a patient on chronic corticosteroids.

DIFFERENTIAL DIAGNOSIS

The differential diagnosis includes the following: other autoimmune diseases (MCTD, drug-induced lupus, autoimmune hepatitis, Evan syndrome, primary antiphospholipid antibody syndrome, primary Sjögren syndrome, and so on); malignancy; systemic vasculitis; juvenile idiopathic arthritis (systemic); or systemic viral infection (*Table 15*) (Woo *et al.* 2007).

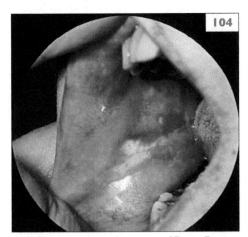

104

104 Oral ulceration (courtesy of Dawn Davis, MD, Mayo Clinic).

Table 14
Active and chronic glomerular lesions (adapted from Weening *et al.* 2004)

Active lesions

Endocapillary hypercellularity with or without leukocyte infiltration and with substantial luminal reduction

Karyorrhexis

Fibrinoid necrosis

Rupture of glomerular basement membrane

Crescents, cellular or fibrocellular

Subendothelial deposits identifiable by light microscopy (wireloops)

Intraluminal immune aggregates (hyaline thrombi)

Chronic lesions

Glomerular sclerosis (segmental, global)

Fibrous adhesions

Fibrous crescents

Table 15
Differential diagnosis for systemic lupus erythematosus (adapted from Woo *et al.* 2007)

Disease category	Common features	Differences
Other autoimmune diseases (MCTD, drug-induced lupus, autoimmune hepatitis, Evan syndrome, primary antiphospholipid antibody syndrome, primary Sjögren syndrome, and so on)	Fever, cytopenia, fatigue, rash	Lack of specific autoantibodies (dsDNA, Smith), specific features unique to specific diseases (e.g. Gottron papules in juvenile dermatomyositis)
Malignancy	Fever, cytopenia, fatigue, pain, lymphadenopathy, hepatosplenomegaly	Night pain, bone tenderness, normal complement, no urinary changes
Systemic vasculitis	Fever, fatigue, rash	Nodules, calf pain, positive ANCA, bruits
Juvenile idiopathic arthritis (systemic)	Arthritis, fatigue, fever, rash, lymphadenopathy, marked anemia	Lack of specific autoantibodies, normal complements, no major organ dysfunction
Systemic viral infection	Fever, lymphadenopathy, hepatosplenomegaly, cytopenias	Lack of specific autoantibodies, normal complements

PROGNOSIS

The natural history of lupus is characterized by a widely variable and unpredictable clinical course with periods of flare and quiescence. Left untreated, SLE often results in progressive deterioration with a significant fatality rate. However, survival in pediatric SLE has dramatically improved over the last 20 years, the result of earlier and more accurate diagnosis, recognition of mild forms of disease, and better approaches to treatments (Ravelli *et al.* 2005). In terms of long-term survival for all lupus patients in the 2000s, the 5-year survival rate approaches 100% and the 10-year survival rate is close to 90%. However, these numbers reflect all lupus patients and are not specific to lupus patients with a particular organ system disease.

Other important lupus outcome measures include disease activity, cumulative organ damage, and functional health status. Several studies have shown that cumulative organ damage is common in patients with pediatric-onset SLE, with a frequency of damage of 50.5–61% (Ravelli *et al.* 2005). Most of the damage occurs in the musculoskeletal, renal, and neuropsychiatric systems, although the current damage index does not take into account pediatric-specific issues such as growth retardation, pubertal development, and the regenerative ability of children to recover and reverse some forms of damage. The outcome is worse in patients with proliferative renal disease and/or CNS disease, and both are the leading causes of death in SLE after infectious causes.

Unfortunately, studies have also shown that patients with pediatric-onset SLE have poorer health-related quality of life and lower socio–economic status compared with their healthy peers (Ravelli *et al.* 2005). Patients with childhood-onset SLE are living longer, but are subsequently dealing with the burden of chronic disease and treatment-associated morbidities, which greatly impact their physical, psychological, and financial wellbeing. Patients with pediatric SLE are entering into adult life challenged with the sequelae of disease activity, permanent organ damage, medication toxicity, and other comorbidities such as recurrent infections, accelerated atherosclerosis, osteoporosis and/or avascular necrosis, hypertension, infertility, and increased risk of malignancies.

MANAGEMENT

There is a wide range of disease severity and it is crucial to tailor specific treatment to the degree of organ system involvement to prevent treatment-related toxicities. Most of the lupus treatments used in children have been extrapolated from adult clinical trial data, which may not be completely applicable. Special considerations need to be made regarding the growth and development of children on chronic, often aggressive, medications. Compliance issues in the adolescent period can lead to severe consequences and poor outcomes. Treatment for pediatric SLE can be roughly divided into mild, moderate, and severe categories. Patients with childhood-onset SLE require treatment with high-dose corticosteroid (Tucker *et al.* 1995) and other immunosuppressive agents more often than adults (Brunner *et al.* 2002). Patients with APL antibody syndrome may require prophylaxis with aspirin or other anticoagulation. The management of SLE is outlined in the table (*Table 16*).

COMPLICATIONS

Since SLE is a multisystem disease, many organs have the potential to be damaged. Decreased cognitive function, seizures, and paralysis are examples of possible neurologic complications. Renal failure and hypertension may be the result of renal involvement. The arthritis is not destructive. Bleeding can occur from severe thrombocytopenia. Opportunistic infections may occur from leukopenia. Complications of medical therapies such as gastritis associated with NSAIDs, infections associated with immunosuppressive medications, and bone disease related to corticosteroids may occur.

Table 16
Management principles for systemic lupus erythematosus

	Characteristics	Treatment
Mild lupus	No renal or other major organ system involvement. Presence of rashes, arthralgias and/or arthritis, leukopenia, anemia, fever, and fatigue	NSAIDs; low-dose corticosteroids (prednisone 0.5 mg/kg per day); antimalarials (hydroxychloroquine); low-dose methotrexate (0.5 mg/kg per week)
Moderate lupus	Mild disease with mild organ system involvement such as minor pericarditis, pneumonitis, hemolytic anemia, thrombocytopenia, mild renal disease, and mild CNS disease	NSAIDs; medium-dose corticosteroids (prednisone 1–2 mg/kg per day); antimalarials; low-dose; methotrexate; azathioprine; mycophenolate mofetil
Severe lupus	Life-threatening, organ system abnormalities, such as severe hemolytic anemia, CNS disease, lupus nephritis, and lupus crisis	High, often pulse-dose corticosteroids (2–3 mg/kg per day or pulse dose 30 mg/kg per day i.v.) in combination with immunosuppressives: cyclophosphamide, azathioprine, methotrexate, cyclosporine, mycophenolate mofetil, or rituximab. In certain situations: plasmapheresis, IVIG, and anticoagulation. Dialysis and renal transplantation in patients with end-stage renal disease

Mixed connective tissue disease

DEFINITION
Some children present with signs and symptoms characteristic of two or more major rheumatic disorders, including JIA, SLE, juvenile dermatomyositis, and/or systemic sclerosis. These children may be classified as having mixed connective tissue disease (MCTD), one of the least common disorders in pediatric rheumatology. Children with MCTD often have very high titers of antibodies to RNP. Three sets of classification criteria for MCTD are widely used that include a variety of clinical features. Kasukawa criteria are used most frequently in the pediatric setting (*Table 17*) (Kasukawa 1987).

EPIDEMIOLOGY AND ETIOLOGY
MCTD is one of the rarest pediatric rheumatology diseases, with a frequency of 0.3% in the US rheumatology database (Black & Isenberg 1992). Although pediatric presentations make up 23% of all cases of MCTD, one study estimated 0.6% prevalence of all pediatric rheumatologic patients (Mier *et al.* 2005). Median age at onset is 11 years, ranging from 4 years to 16 years. MCTD is three times more common in girls than in boys (Black & Isenberg 1992). The presence of haplotypes HLA-DR4 and HLA-DR2 is associated with MCTD. However, given that MCTD is a disease with overlapping features of other autoimmune diseases, the following associations have also been reported: HLA-DR2 and HLA-DR3 (associated with SLE); HLA-DR5 (associated with systemic sclerosis); and HLA-DR3 (associated with dermatomyositis) (Smolen & Steiner 1998).

CLINICAL HISTORY
Because of the wide range of symptoms encompassed by this disease, there are several variations reported for clinical manifestations: (1) SLE-like features; (2) scleroderma-like features; and (3) myositis-like features (*Table 18*). Clinical features of MCTD have included the following (Black & Isenberg 1992, Cassidy & Petty 2005, Michels 1997, Mier *et al.* 2005, Mukerji & Hardin 1993, Smolen & Steiner 1998, Tiddens *et al.* 1993, Yokota 1993):
- Constitutional – fatigue, weight loss.
- Musculoskeletal – arthralgias are common; myalgias are present mostly at disease onset.

Table 17
Kasukawa's criteria for mixed connective tissue disease

Patients must meet all three of the following criteria to be diagnosed with MCTD:
- Raynaud phenomenon or swollen fingers or hands or both
- Anti-RNP antibody positivity
- At least one abnormal finding from two or more of the following categories:
- Signs or symptoms of SLE (polyarthritis, facial rash, serositis, lymphadenopathy, leukopenia, or thrombocytopenia)
- Signs or symptoms of scleroderma (sclerodactyly, pulmonary fibrosis, vital capacity <80% of normal, carbon monoxide diffusion <70% of normal, decreased esophageal motility)
- Signs or symptoms of dermatomyositis (muscle weakness, elevated creatinine kinase, EMG abnormalities)

Table 18
Frequencies of mixed connective tissue disease manifestations at presentation and course

Disease manifestation	At presentation (%)	Disease course (%)
SLE like	6	18
Scleroderma like	15	26
Myositis like	32	40

n = 34 patients

- Cardiovascular – Raynaud phenomenon is one of the most common initial signs. Pericarditis, vasculitis, and hypertension have all been described.
- Gastrointestinal – dysphagia can occur secondary to abnormal esophageal and bowel motility.
- Neurologic – trigeminal neuropathy is the most frequent neurologic finding (25% in adults). Transverse myelopathy, seizures, and psychosis have also been reported.
- Pulmonary – signs of interstitial disease, pulmonary hypertension and serositis have also been reported.

- Renal – glomerulonephritis and renal insufficiency can occur.
- Glandular – Sjögren syndrome reported in three-quarters of children but xerostomia, parotid swelling, and parotitis are present in only 15–20%.

PHYSICAL EXAMINATION

Clinical features of MCTD have included the following (Black & Isenberg 1992, Cassidy & Petty 2005, Michels 1997, Mier *et al.* 2005, Mukerji & Hardin 1993, Smolen & Steiner 1998, Tiddens *et al.* 1993, Yokota 1993):

- Constitutional – weight loss.
- Musculoskeletal – non-erosive polyarthritis is possible. Inflammatory muscle disease with muscle weakness, mostly at disease onset.
- Dermatologic – sclerodermatous skin changes, hand edema (**105**), and nailfold capillary abnormalities (**106**). Digital ulcerations, subcutaneous nodules (**107**), calcinosis (**108**), telangiectasias, and photosensitivity can occur. One-third of patients complain of malar rash similar to SLE, and another third of rash similar to juvenile dermatomyositis (JDM), including heliotrope rash and/or Gottron papules.

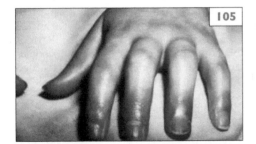

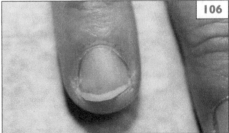

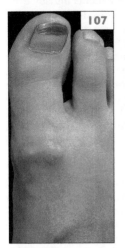

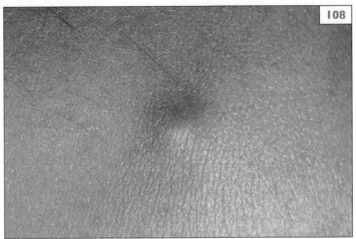

105–108 Hand edema and MCTD (**105**); nailfold capillary changes in MCTD (courtesy of David Fiorentino, MD, Stanford University) (**106**); subcutaneous nodules in a patient with MCTD (**107**); calcinosis and MCTD (**108**).

- Cardiovascular – Raynaud phenomenon is one of the most common initial signs. Pericarditis, vasculitis, and hypertension have all been described.
- Gastrointestinal – hepatomegaly has also been described.
- Neurologic – trigeminal neuropathy is the most frequent neurologic finding (25% in adults). Transverse myelopathy, seizures, and psychosis have also been reported.
- Pulmonary – findings of interstitial lung disease and pulmonary hypertension are the two most common and dangerous manifestations of pulmonary involvement in MCTD. Serositis has also been reported.
- Hematologic – splenomegaly can occur.
- Renal – glomerulonephritis and renal insufficiency can occur.
- Glandular – parotid swelling, and parotitis are present in only 15–20%.

LABORATORY
Most children with MCTD have ANAs and antibodies to RNP. Additional serologies that could be obtained include those more specific for particular rheumatologic diseases, such as: (1) dsDNA and anti-Smith antibodies for SLE; (2) ACA and anti-Scl-70 antibodies for scleroderma; and (3) RF for JIA. The arthritis of MCTD is often associated with a positive RF and can be present in two-thirds of children with MCTD. Children with MCTD may have more frequent and severe renal disease than adults, warranting periodic urine analyses. Children with MCTD also may have more hematologic complications such as thrombocytopenia than adults, and screening CBCs should be obtained regularly (Mier *et al.* 2005).

IMAGING
Plain films may be useful to evaluate the extent of arthritis (**109, 110**), although erosive bone disease in MCTD is rare. A chest rediograph may be helpful in evaluating for possible cardiopulmonary disease. Children with MCTD have less pulmonary hypertension than adults, but a baseline cardiac echocardiogram and/or pulmonary function test with D_{LCO} may be indicated in a child with concerning symptoms. A high-resolution chest CT scan may be indicated if there is concern for pulmonary fibrosis. An upper GI series with small bowel follow-through or swallow study may be useful in evaluating for esophageal or GI dysmotility or strictures.

DIFFERENTIAL DIAGNOSIS
Given the amount of overlap MCTD has with other rheumatologic diseases, it is important to ensure that the patient does not actually have an unusual presentation of a particular connective tissue disease, such as SLE, juvenile idiopathic arthritis, dermatomyositis, polymyositis, systemic sclerosis, localized scleroderma, or Sjögren disease.

PROGNOSIS
There exists the possibility of clinical evolution of MCTD into a disease that better satisfies another connective tissue disorder, such as lupus, scleroderma, or dermatomyositis; therefore, heightened awareness is needed when treating a patient with MCTD. The serologic profile of patients with MCTD may also be somewhat prognostic. Some studies have noted associations between anti-Smith and renal disease, while other studies have noted associations between anti-RNP and Raynaud phenomenon, myositis, esophageal dysmotility, and pulmonary fibrosis. A meta-analysis reported that remissions occurred in 3–27% of children. Raynaud phenomenon and scleroderma-like skin changes were the most common finding, reported in up to 86% of children (Michels 1997). Another study showed that more than 50% of patients initially diagnosed with MCTD showed features more consistent with progressive systemic sclerosis after 5 years (Mukerji & Hardin 1993). Renal disease was uncommon but was the cause of the only two disease-related deaths in the study. Pulmonary hypertension and CNS disease have been shown to be persistent, possibly relaying worse prognosis (Kasukawa 1987). The annual disease-specific mortality in pediatric MCTD is reported to be 3–4 per 1000 patients (Mier *et al.* 2005).

MANAGEMENT
MCTD was initially characterized as a disorder with an excellent initial response to glucocorticoid therapy; however, therapy is directed at the specific symptoms of the child, such as arthritis, cutaneous disease, or other organ involvement. Tiddens *et al.* reported the use of NSAIDs in 78%, corticosteroids in 71%, and hydroxy-

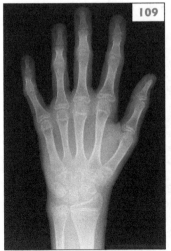
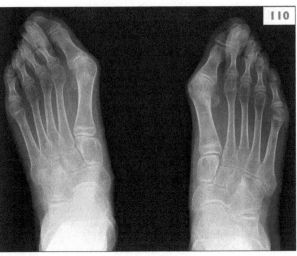

109, 110 Radiograph of patient with MCTD, showing patient's hands with diffuse erosive arthritis with joint space narrowing (**109**); radiograph of patient with MCTD showing erosions from active arthritis (**110**).

chloroquine in 50% in their series of 14 patients (Tiddens *et al.* 1993). Other immunosuppressive medications used to treat children with MCTD include methotrexate, mycophenolate mofetil, azathioprine, cyclosporine, cyclophosphamide, etanercept, and infliximab (Cimaz *et al.* 2003). Calcium channel blockers such as amlodipine and nifedipine and topical nitropaste can be used for complaints of Raynaud phenomenon.

COMPLICATIONS
Since MCTD is an 'overlap' condition with features of several other connective tissue diseases, many organs have the potenial to be damaged. Myocardial involvement can lead to cardiac dysfunction. Pulmonary fibrosis may occur after interstitial lung disease. Digital ischemia may also occur. Opportunistic infections can occur from severe skin changes. The arthritis is usually not destructive. Complications of medical therapies such as gastritis associated with NSAIDs, infections associated with immunosuppressive medications, and bone disease related to corticosteroids may occur.

Neonatal lupus syndrome

DEFINITION

Neonatal lupus syndrome (NLS) is a passively acquired autoimmune disease that occurs in neonates born to mothers who have specific autoantibodies. These autoantibodies pass through the placenta and can cause neonatal organ damage including to the skin, liver, brain, heart, blood vessels, and blood elements.

EPIDEMIOLOGY AND ETIOLOGY

In women with SSA/Ro antibodies, 27% of infants develop hematologic abnormalities, 26% develop liver enzyme elevation, 16% develop cutaneous lesions, and 1.6% develop complete congenital heart block (Cimaz *et al.* 2003). Half of infants with NLS have mothers who are clinically well.

NLS results from transplacental passage of autoantibodies which target fetal and neonatal tissues for immune destruction. Implicated autoantibodies include anti-SSA, anti-SSB, and anti-RNP antibodies (Buyon *et al.* 1994). The characteristic pathologic findings reveal inflammatory cell infiltrates and deposition of immunoglobulin, complement, and fibrin in the various organs and tissues.

CLINICAL HISTORY

Since NLS presents in the newborn, most of the relevant history is maternal, such as the presence of a connective tissue disorder such as SLE or Sjögren syndrome. These connective tissue disorders are characterized by the presence of autoantibodies that could cross the placenta perinatally. The presence of bradycardia, cytopenias, or characteristic skin lesions in a newborn also prompts an evaluation for NLS. The fetal bradycardia could be detected *in utero* prior to delivery.

PHYSICAL EXAMINATION

Each of the following manifestations can occur in isolation or in combination:

- Skin – the classic NLS rash is characterized by round or elliptical, erythematous, papulosquamous lesions with a fine scale and central clearing (**111**). Annular erythema (**112**), bullous lesions on the soles and palms, and facial telangiectasias have also been described. Lesions typically involve the face and scalp, but are also found on the neck, trunk, extremities, and intertriginous areas. A raccoon-eye rash is common, whereas the malar rash is rarely seen. The rash may be be present at birth but more commonly develops within the first few months of life. Lesions can develop at any time up to 6 months of age, and can be exacerbated by sunlight or phototherapy. The rash spontaneously resolves by 6–8 months as maternal autoantibodies disappear from the infant's circulation. Residual dyspigmentation and atrophy are rare.

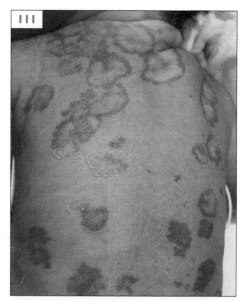

111 Newborn with neonatal lupus rash.

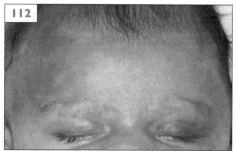

112 Neonatal lupus rash.

- Cardiac – the most severe and life-threatening complication is congenital heart block (CHB). CHB occurs in 1 in 14,000 live births and at least 90% of these cases are due to transplacental passage of maternal autoantibodies (Buyon et al. 1998). The incidence of heart block in infants born to mothers who have anti-SSA or anti-SSB antibodies is 1–2%, and the recurrence rate in subsequent pregnancies is 16–18% (Brucato et al. 2002, Buyon et al. 1998, Cimaz et al. 2003). Complete CHB causes significant morbidity and mortality, with 65% of surviving neonates ultimately requiring pacemakers (Buyon et al. 1998). Incomplete heart block can progress to higher degrees of block years after the postnatal period (Askanase et al. 2002). Additional ECG abnormalities have been reported including transient sinus bradycardia, QT interval prolongations, and Wolff–Parkinson–White syndrome (Askanase et al. 2002). Ventricular endocardial fibroelastosis can present prenatally or postnatally in the first year of life.
- Hematologic manifestations – thrombocytopenia and anemia are the most common hematologic manifestations and typically worsen in the first days after birth and resolve after disappearance of maternal autoantibodies. Cases of neutropenia, transient pancytopenia, aplastic anemia, hemolytic anemia, and thrombosis have also been reported.
- Liver – the primary manifestations are transaminitis, cholestasis, and hepatosplenomegaly. The two most common presentations of NLS liver disease are: (1) direct hyperbilirubinemia with mild or no transaminitis occurring in the first few weeks after birth, and (2) mild transaminitis occurring at 2–3 months of age (Lee et al. 2002). Most infants have spontaneous resolution of liver abnormalities by 6 months after clearance of maternal autoantibodies. Severe perinatal hepatic dysfunction, often with the phenotype of neonatal iron storage disease, suggests a poor prognosis and warrants treatment with corticosteroids (Frankovich et al. 2008).
- Central nervous system – cerebral hypomyelination, hydrocephalus, and macrocephaly are the most common reported findings (Boros et al. 2007, Prendiville et al. 2003). Cerebral dysmaturation and vasculopathy affecting the blood vessels that supply the basal ganglia and germinal matrix are also reported (Frankovich et al. 2008). Rarely, infants with NLS can have hypotonia, seizures, developmental delay, and feeding difficulty (Frankovich et al. 2008).
- Other manifestations – rhizomelic chondrodysplasia has been reported (Shanske et al. 2007). Pneumonitis, pulmonary capillaritis, glomerulonephritis, and nephrotic syndrome are rare manifestations of NLS and may be suggestive of infantile primary SLE.

LABORATORY

Evaluation for maternal autoantibodies should be undertaken if any of the previously described manifestations are present in the neonate without a clear cause. The initial screening can be done using maternal serum or cord blood. A complete evaluation for congenital infection should be pursued simultaneously since congenital infections mimic NLS and require prompt antibiotic therapy. The initial maternal antibody screen should include ANA, anti-SSA antibody, and anti-SSB antibody. Blood counts, liver function tests, and thyroid hormone levels should be evaluated in all infants born to mothers with autoimmune diseases and asymptomatic mothers with implicated autoantibodies.

IMAGING

If maternal autoantibodies are found, fetal cardiac echocardiography should be done to evaluate for evidence of heart block.

DIFFERENTIAL DIAGNOSIS

Congenital infections can cause hepatitis, basal ganglia calcifications, and hematologic abnormalities which are similar in presentation to NLS. Neonatal iron storage disease and giant cell hepatitis have similar liver pathology and presentation. Peroxisomal disorders can also present with rhizomelic chondrodysplasia.

PROGNOSIS

Most manifestations resolve spontaneously by 6 months of age after clearance of maternal antibodies. Permanent sequelae can occur when inflammation is extensive (skin, liver, or bone marrow) or when vulnerable tissues are involved (cardiac conduction system and small end-organ blood vessels). Maternal disease activity during pregnancy predicts worse outcomes. High titers of maternal SSA antibodies and the presence of maternal thyroid disease increase the risk of NLS complications. Future development of an autoimmune disease in early childhood warrants long-term follow-up of infants with NLS (Martin et al. 2002).

MANAGEMENT

All pregnant women with autoimmune symptoms should undergo early first-trimester screening of implicated antibodies. Women found to have positive anti-SSA and anti-SSB should be considered at high risk for development of CHB in the fetus. Current recommendations are to monitor the fetal PR interval by echocardiogram weekly between 16 and 26 weeks' gestation, and biweekly between 26 and 32 weeks. For cardiac involvement, maternal oral dexamethasone therapy and IVIG *in utero* have been used but efficacy and risks are still questionable. Sympathomimetics are used for severe intrauterine and postnatal bradycardia until a pacemaker can be placed. Corticosteroids are recommended for active carditis postnatally. In cases of severe symptomatic fetal thrombocytopenia and anemia, IVIG and corticosteroids have been used. Corticosteroids are also used for severe or persistent liver involvement.

In most cases, affected neonates present with an isolated manifestation of NLS, although multiorgan dysfunction can occur. The most common multiorgan presentation of NLS is a sick preterm infant who has anemia, thrombocytopenia, liver dysfunction, and respiratory failure. In addition to the standard evaluation for congenital infection, a timely evaluation for NLS, including ECG and maternal autoantibody profiles, may facilitate diagnosis. In addition, maternal thyroid and APL antibodies may be measured and a careful neurologic examination undertaken.

COMPLICATIONS

The primary complication from NLS is permanent damage to the neonatal cardiac conduction system. There is risk for bleeding and infection with the associated cytopenias.

Cutaneous lupus erythematosus

DEFINITION

Cutaneous lupus erythematosus (CLE) is a heterogeneous group of connective tissue diseases represented by skin manifestations. The skin lesions are characterized by the presence or absence of interface dermatitis and the presence or absence of scarring. There are three categories based on Gilliam's classification system (Gilliam & Sontheimer 1981).

EPIDEMIOLOGY AND ETIOLOGY

CLE is thought to occur two to three times more frequently than SLE with the most common age between 20 and 40 years. There exists a female:male predominance of 3–6:1 depending on the subtype of CLE (Tebbe & Orfanos 1997). In multiple studies of CLE patients, age of onset varied from 8 years to 84 years of age with only around 3% presenting younger than 20 years of age. African–Americans tended to have a higher prevalence of chronic CLE than whites (Tebbe & Orfanos 1997).

The etiology for CLE is thought to be multifactoral, with genetic predisposition, environmental factors, and host immune factors all contributing. Genetic associations have been reported of subacute SCL (SCLE) with C2 and C4 deficiencies, HLA-B8, HLA-DR3, HLA-DRw52, HLA-DQ1, and HLA-DQ2; associations of acute CLE (ACLE) with HLA-DR2 and HLA-DR3; and associations of chronic CLE (CCLE) with C1q, C3, C5 deficiencies (Patel & Werth 2002). Complement deficiencies are thought to cause failure of the clearance of apoptotic cells, which in turn causes increased immunologic stimulation. The cytokines that have been implicated in CCLE include IL-2 and interferon-γ, with CD45RA+ T cells being the prevailing inflammatory cells. It has been reported that 65–70% of CLE patients will have exacerbating or aggravating skin reactions when exposed to UVA and UVB light. This reaction can be delayed for up to months after the exposure. It is hypothesized that keratinocyte-induced apoptosis by antibody-mediated cellular cytotoxicity reactions causes autoantibody production. Drugs such as hydrochlorothiazide, calcium channel blockers, angiotensin-converting enzyme inhibitors, and anti-TNF antagonists, certain viruses such as Epstein–Barr virus, cytomegalovirus, and human immunodeficiency virus, long-term silica exposure, and smoking have been implicated in CLE induction (Patel & Werth 2002).

CLINICAL HISTORY

- Acute cutaneous lupus erythematosus – photosensitivity is a primary feature. Alopecia can also develop.
- Subacute cutaneous lupus erythematosus – photosensitivity is also prominent.
- Chronic cutaneous lupus erythematosus – as with ACLE, and SCLE, photosensitivity occurs. Unlike ACLE and SCLE, CCLE can result in scarring. CCLE is the most common subtype of CLE. CCLE can be associated with systemic symptoms such as arthritis and arthralgias (15–20%). CCLE can present in a variety of ways: discoid lupus erythematosus (DLE) (localized and generalized), hypertrophic LE, lupus panniculitis, and mucosal DLE. The most common type is DLE (**113a, 113b**), which has sharply demarcated scaly erythematous papules or plaques that can extend into the follicles. Patients with localized DLE (>50% of CCLE) have lesions that involve only the neck and head as well as fewer manifestations of systemic diseases. Patients with widespread DLE (5–10% of CCLE) called DLE-SLE may progress to systemic disease within 1–3 years. DLE lesions can also develop into squamous cell carcinoma.

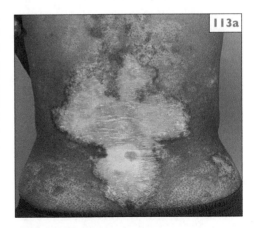

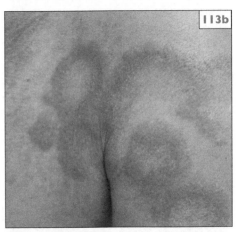

113a, 113b DLE rash (courtesy of Dawn Davis, MD, Mayo Clinic) (**113a**); DLE rash on the arm and chest (**113b**).

PHYSICAL EXAMINATION

- Acute cutaneous lupus erythematosus – non-scarring lesions with an intermittent course that usually involves the face, chest, shoulders, and extensor surfaces of the arm and hand. There can be an associated superficial ulceration of nasal and oral mucosa. The most common localized ACLE rash is the classic malar or butterfly rash. The most generalized ACLE rash is photosensitive lupus dermatitis. Furthermore, diffuse hair thinning, lupus hair, telangiectasias, and proximal nailfold erythema have been reported.

- Subacute cutaneous lupus erythematosus – usually non-scarring lesions with an intermittent course that commonly involves the face and neck (**114**). It usually presents as a papulosquamous or annular polycyclic eruption. The lesions from SCLE can have a psoriasis-type or pityriasis look to them. In addition, malar eruption, livedo reticularis, periungal telangiectasias, and generalized poikiloderma have been reported.
- Chronic cutaneous lupus erythematosus – more generalized skin lesions that can result in scarring, atrophy, and follicular plugging.

LABORATORY

All lab results associated with SLE can also occur with CLE (more with ACLE and less with CCLE). However, association with SLE serology is neither diagnostic nor exclusionary. The following laboratory results have been reported in CLE: anti-dsDNA antibody (SCLE 5–30%, ACLE 60–80%), anti-SSA antibodies (SCLE 90%), anti-Sm antibodies, elevated ESR, low complements (C3, C4, CH50), hematologic abnormalities (anemia, leukopenia, thrombocytopenia), and hypergammaglobulinemia. The lupus band test, now rarely used, may reveal immunoglobulin and/or complement deposition at the dermal–epidermal junction (SCLE 60%, DLE 90%) (Callen 2006).

IMAGING

None is helpful unless organ system involvement is present.

DIFFERENTIAL DIAGNOSIS

- **ACLE** – drug eruptions, drug-induced photosensitivity, dermatomyositis, bullous lesions of toxic epidural necrolysis.
- **SCLE** – urticarial vasculitis and other cutaneous vasculitic syndromes; annular SCLE often needs to be differentiated from erythema annulare centrifugum, and papulosquamous SCLE from lichen planus, psoriasis, and/or dermatomyositis.
- **CCLE** – papulosquamous diseases and chronic eczema in DLE; non-melanoma skin cancers, keratoacanthomas, and warts.

PROGNOSIS

Overall, it appears that patients with isolated CLE have a better prognosis than patients with SLE; however, severe life-threatening systemic complications can occur in CLE patients. Renal and CNS involvement have been reported (Tebbe & Orfanos 1997). The extent of skin involvement may predict disease severity, with less systemic involvement in patients with skin lesions limited to the face or scalp (Tebbe & Orfanos 1997). Disease activity of CLE can be variable but has been reported to persist up to 41 years (Tebbe & Orfanos 1997). One study showed that CLE patients with signs of nephropathy, arthralgias, and high-titer ANAs (>1:320) should be carefully monitored for transition into SLE (Tebbe & Orfanos 1997). Patients with ACLE have a high risk (up to 100%) of developing SLE whereas patients with SCLE have a much lower risk (about 10%) of developing SLE. With regard to CCLE, patients with localized DLE have a 5% risk of developing SLE while patients with diffuse DLE have about a 20% risk in developing SLE.

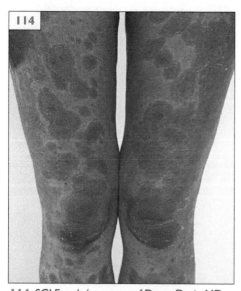

114 SCLE rash (courtesy of Dawn Davis, MD, Mayo Clinic).

MANAGEMENT

The main goals of management are to prevent lesion progression, provide counseling about systemic disease surveillance, and improve physical appearance. Patient education is very important as many factors are known to flare and exacerbate the disease; it consists of avoidance of certain drugs associated with CLE, taking sun- and heat-protective measures, and refraining from smoking. Patients should be aware that there exists the possibility of transition to SLE and they should be appropriately screened with routine blood and urine tests.

Localized CLE can be treated with varying potency topical steroids depending on the location of the lesions, with lower potency for facial lesions and higher potency for the palms and soles. Intralesional steroids and lasers have been reported to treat localized CLE. Other non-steroidal topical agents used include: retinoids (i.e. tretinoin); immunomodulators (i.e. tacrolimus 0.1%); calcipotriene; and imiquimod. Systemic treatment of CLE includes the use of antimalarials such as hydroxychloroquine as a first-line agent. In more diffuse cases, systemic corticosteroids, antibiotics (i.e. dapsone, cefuroxime axetil, sulfasalazine, and clofazimine), auranofin (oral gold effective in SCLE), thalidomide, and oral phenytoin have been used. Immunosuppressive agents such as azathioprine, methotrexate, mycophenolate mofetil, cyclosporine, and cyclophosphamide have been reported for refractory cases. The use of biologics is limited with the concern that such drugs can lead to the development of drug-induced SLE and SCLE (Callen 2006, Patel & Werth 2002).

COMPLICATIONS

One of the primary complications of the cutaneous forms of lupus is the conversion to SLE. Skin cancers may also develop.

CHAPTER 5

Idiopathic inflammatory myopathies

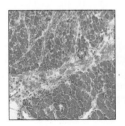
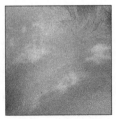
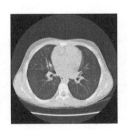
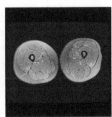

The juvenile inflammatory myopathies are systemic, autoimmune inflammatory muscle disorders that occur in children younger than 18 years of age. Three general types commonly seen in pediatric rheumatology are juvenile dermatomyositis, juvenile polymyositis, and postinfectious myositis.

Juvenile dermatomyositis

DEFINITION

Juvenile dermatomyositis (JDM) is an inflammatory vasculopathy that affects primarily the skin and the skeletal muscles. JDM represents 20% of all inflammatory myositis and is the most common inflammatory myopathy in children. Classic findings are Gottron rash and papules, heliotrope rash, calcinosis cutis, and symmetric, proximal muscle weakness. Diagnosis is made by Bohan and Peter (1975a): a characteristic rash, proximal muscle weakness, elevated muscle enzymes, EMG results of polyphasic, low-amplitude motor unit potentials with insertional irritability and fibrillations, and muscle biopsy with inflammation and/or vasculitis. Skin findings with three other features are necessary to make the diagnosis (*Table 19*).

Table 19
Clinical criteria for juvenile dermatomyositis

Characteristic skin findings
   Gottron papules
   Erythematous rash
   Periungual erythema and telangiectasis
   Alopecia
   Calcinosis

Characteristic muscle findings
   Symmetric proximal weakness
   Elevation of muscle enzymes
   Typical EMG pattern
   Vasculitis and/or inflammation on muscle biopsy

EPIDEMIOLOGY AND ETIOLOGY

The estimated annual incidence in whites is 3.4 cases per million; there is a higher incidence in Hispanics and African–Americans. Females are affected more often than males. The median age of onset is approximately 7 years with a median delay to diagnosis of 3–4 months.

The etiology is not completely understood. The innate and adaptive immune systems and environmental factors may trigger JDM in a genetically susceptible host. Seasonal clustering of JDM in the spring months suggests that environmental agents play an important role in disease onset. An upper respiratory infection may be seen in 56% of patients with JDM 3 months before onset of symptoms as per data collected by the National Juvenile Dermatomyositis Registry. The relationships to infectious agents associated with development of JDM such as Coxsackie B virus, adenovirus, echovirus, hepatitis B, toxoplasmosis, influenza, parvovirus B19, enterovirus, *Mycobacteria pneumoniae*, and *Streptococcus* spp. are all indirect. Molecular mimicry may play a causative role. However, the evidence is inconclusive as there has not been viral or bacterial DNA found in muscle biopsy specimens. Non-infectious agents such as exposure to UV light and bone marrow transplantation as in a graft-versus-host paradigm are also hypothesized to be factors in JDM (*Table 20*).

The pathogenesis of JDM involves the innate and adaptive immune system with the humoral and cell-mediated pathways causing vascular and muscle damage. There is increased expression of major histocompatibility complex class I and II. Autoantibodies against endothelial antigens, currently unknown, may produce vascular injury leading to ischemia and muscle damage. An inflammatory lymphocytic infiltrate involving CD4+ T cells, B cells, plasmacytoid dendritic cells, and macrophages is present in the muscles and the skin. These cells are arranged in a perivascular and perifascicular distribution (**115**). There is perifascicular atrophy of type I and type II fibers. Swelling and occlusion of the capillary lumen with muscle degeneration and regeneration are characteristic findings. Infarcts and necrosis of muscle fibers can occur in the fascicle. Immune complex deposition with membrane attack complexes produces muscle inflammation.

Table 20
Environmental causes of myositis

Agents	Observations
Infectious	
Coxsackie virus	Antibodies to Coxsackie B viruses noted at onset of JDM compared with controls few in studies
Influenza virus	Seen with acute viral myositis children who subsequently developed JDM
Hepatitis B and C	Myositis development associated after acute illness
Parvovirus	Myositis development associated after acute illness
Echovirus	Myositis seen mainly in children with X-linked hypogammaglobulinemia
Streptococcus spp.	Elevated titers seen in children before onset of myositis
Mycoplasma pneumoniae	Case reports of myositis after pneumonia
Toxoplasmosis	Elevated titers noted before disease onset
Non-infectious	
Drugs	JDM and JPM noted after penicillamine
Vaccines	Agents include MMR, DPT, BCG, hepatitis B several months after vaccination
Bone marrow	JDM and JPM reported after transplantation in a graft-versus-host disease
UV light	JDM seen after excessive sun exposure

CLINICAL HISTORY

Constitutional symptoms may occur 3 months prior to disease onset. Photosensitive rashes can occur coupled with muscle pain and weakness. Thirty percent of children demonstrate a rash at least 3 months prior to muscle weakness; also, 30% of children may experience muscle weakness prior to a rash. Sixty percent of children develop skin and muscle manifestations within 3 months of each other. The child may have difficulty getting out of bed or tire easily in physical education classes or sporting events.

Other symptoms include dysphonia, hoarseness, and melena as a consequence of vasculopathy involving the GI tract. Perforation may occur in up to 5% of patients by occlusion and infarction of the vessels; secondary infection may result as a complication (*Table 21*).

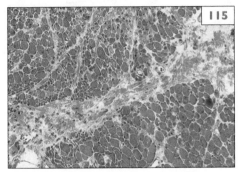

115 Perivascular and perifascicular infiltrates seen in JDM.

Table 21
Clinical presentation of juvenile dermatomyositis

Symptoms	Percentage
Weakness	<100
Rash	100
Muscle pain	72
Fever	65
Swallowing difficulty	45
Abdominal pain	37
Arthritis	36
Calcinosis	22

PHYSICAL EXAMINATION

Skin findings may be prominent and are classic in JDM. The eyelids may be swollen with a heliotrope rash and an overlying scale (**116–118, 119**). A malar rash in a photosensitive distribution and sparing of the nasolabial folds may occur (**120, 121, 122, 123**). Also, patches of erythema with poikilodermatous changes may occur in various areas of the face and the anterior and posterior neck (**124–128**). The 'shawl sign' may be present (**129**).

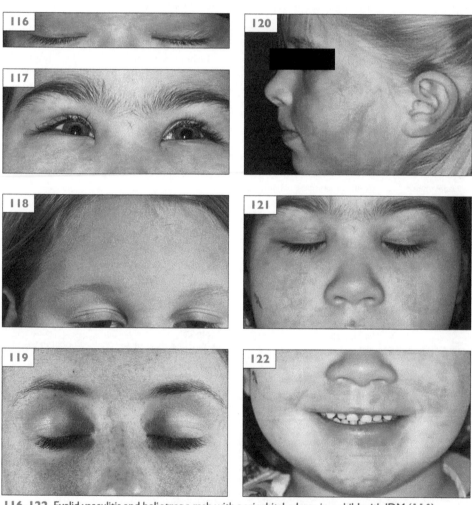

116–122 Eyelid vasculitis and heliotrope rash with periorbital edema in a child with JDM (**116**); a heliotrope rash with periorbital edema in a child with JDM (**117**); facial erythema, scaling and heliotrope rash in a child with JDM (**118**); patchy, erythematous macular rash of the cheeks and upper eyelid in JDM. The erythematous rash spares the perioral region (**119**); patchy, erythematous macular rash of the cheeks and upper eyelid in JDM. The erythemasus rash spares the perioral region (**120**); patchy, erythematous macular rash of the cheeks and upper eyelid and a heliotrope rash in JDM. The erythematous rash spares the perioral region (**121**); patchy, erythematous macular rash with atrophic changes of the cheeks and perioral area in JDM. The erythematous rash spares the perioral region (**122**).

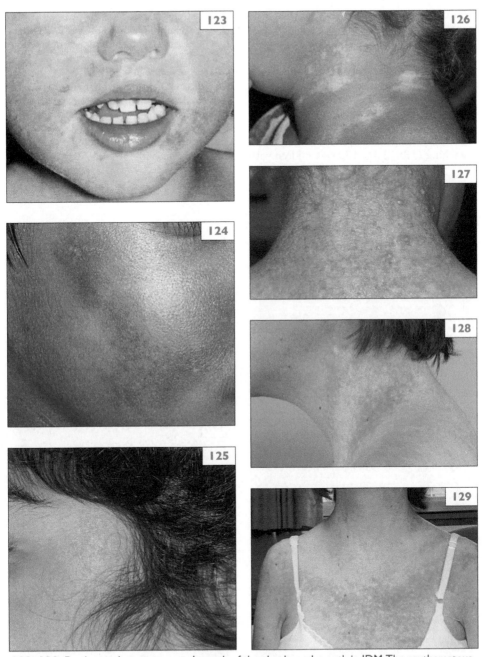

123–129 Patchy, erythematous macular rash of the cheeks and mouth in JDM. The erythematous rash spares the perioral region (**123**); erythematous rash on cheek in JDM (**124**); erythematous rash and atrophic changes on the face in JDM (**125**); erythematous rash with atrophic changes on the neck in JDM (**126**); erythematous rash and calcinosis on posterior neck in JDM (**127**); erythematous rash and calcinosis on neck in JDM (**128**); erythematous rash in a shawl pattern and a V-shaped distribution on the anterior chest, upper arms, and anterior neck in JDM (**129**).

Gottron papules are typical; they are violaceous papules and plaques over bony prominences as in the MCP, PIP, and DIP joints, knees, and ankles (**130, 131, 132a, 132b**). Erythematous, violaceous, scaly plaques may occur over the extensor surfaces of the extremities (**133–135**). Nailfold telangiectasias, periungal erythema, and hypertrophic ragged cuticles may be found with end-row loop capillary loss and bushy loops of capillary dilation and branching (**130, 131, 132a**). Children with inadequately treated disease may demonstrate persistent nailfold changes that may be reflective of disease activity, but not muscle involvement. Finally, mechanic's hands may occur with hyperkeratosis and peeling of the skin over the medial and palmar aspects of the digits. Mechanic's hands can be seen in patients with Jo-1 autoantibody (histidyl-tRNA synthetase) and lung disease. Additional skin findings include panniculitis (**136**) and gum erythema with bleeding (**137**).

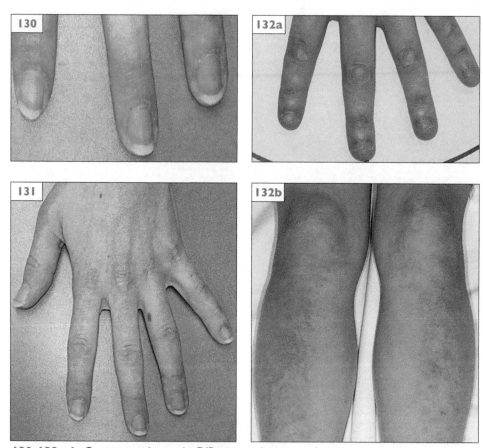

130–132a, b Gottron papules on the DIP joints with periungual capillary loop enlargement and telangiectasias in JDM (**130**); Gottron papules on the MCP and DIP joints with periungual capillary loop enlargement and telangiectasias in JDM (**131**); Gottron papules on the DIP joints, atrophic PIP lesions with periungual capillary loop enlargement and telangiectasias in JDM (**132a**); Gottron rash and extensor erythema on the knees and shins in JDM (**132b**).

133 Gottron papules, erythematous, violaceous papules overlying the elbow joints in a child with JDM.

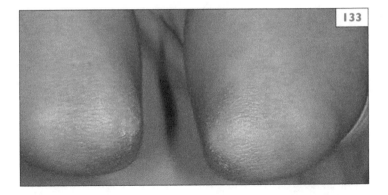

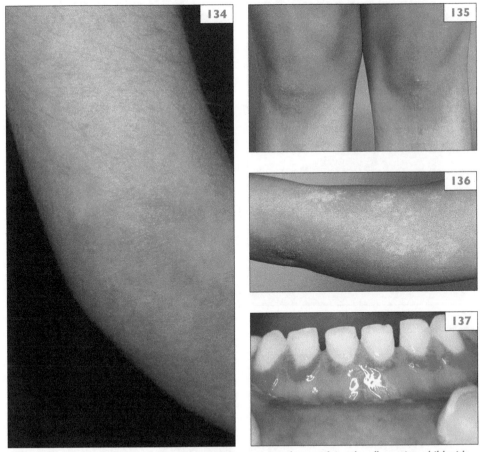

134–137 Gottron papules, erythematous, violaceous papules overlying the elbows in a child with JDM (**134**); Gottron papules, erythematous, violaceous papules overlying the knees in a child with JDM (**135**); panniculitis presenting as firm, painful erythematous lesions (**136**); gum erythema and telangiectasia in JDM (**137**).

Cutaneous vasculitis (**138, 139**) is not uncommon in JDM and may be seen with Raynaud phenomenon as well as cutaneous ulcer, if present, which raises concerns for more severe disease (**140–143**).

Calcinosis has been well described in JDM. The deposits are firm, flesh-colored nodules present over bony prominences, long strips of calcium in the muscle bundles or in the subcutaneous tissue (**144, 145, 145a, 146b**). The most commonly affected areas are the elbows, knees, and extremities (**147, 148**). Calcinosis onset may occur within 3 years of diagnosis, and predictors for devel-

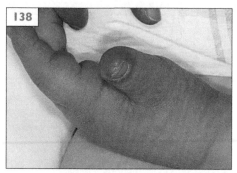

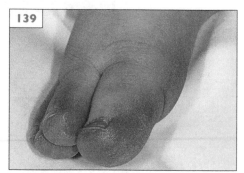

138, 139 Vasculitic skin lesion with severe Raynaud phenomenon in a child with JDM–scleroderma overlap.

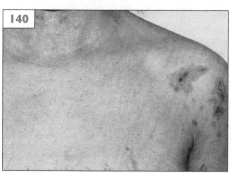

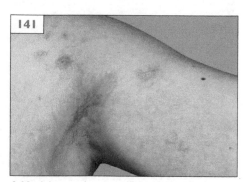

140 A boy with severe JDM with weakness and difficult-to-heal skin ulcerations.

141 A boy with severe JDM with weakness and difficult-to-heal skin ulcerations.

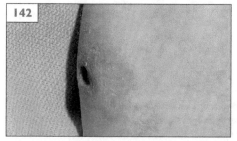

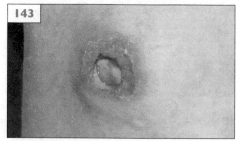

142, 143 A boy with severe JDM with weakness and difficult-to-heal skin ulcerations.

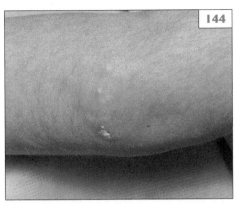

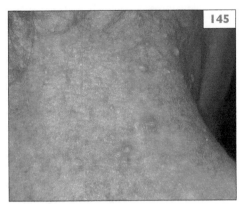

144 Cutaneous calcinosis (courtesy of Lisa Rider MD).

145 Cutaneous calcinosis.

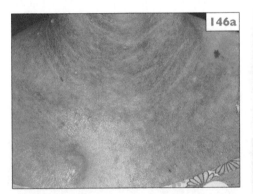

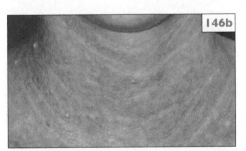

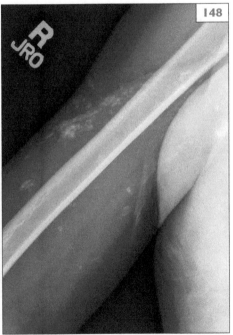

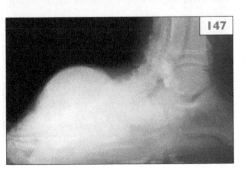

146a, b–148 A girl with erythema and calcinosis on the anterior chest (**146a**); cutaneous calcinosis (**146b**); radiograph of liquified and crystallized calcinosis in the foot of a patient with JDM (**147**); radiograph of the arm of a patient with JDM showing sheet-like calcinosis of the fascia (**148**).

opment include poor clinical response to treatment, insufficient steroid use, and evidence of a severe vasculitis on biopsy.

Lipodystrophy is seen in a subset of JDM, usually those with long-standing and difficult-to-treat disease. Loss of extremity fat (**149**) and an increase in truncal fat, with elevated tryglycerides, alterations of glucose, and insulin metabolism. Poikiloderma is commonly seen associated with lipodystrophy (**150**). Complications such as striae, most commonly from corticosteroid use, may develop (**151**).

Symmetric, proximal muscle weakness is seen in most children, although it may present insidiously. Muscle involvement usually occurs in the deltoids and the quadriceps muscles, or both muscle groups. The child may demonstrate an abnormal Gower maneuver with an inability to rise to a standing position without the use of the arms.

Other organ systems may be commonly involved in JDM – including interstitial lung disease (**152–155**), GI vasculitis, dysphonia, and dysphagia – and less commonly cardiac, ophthalmologic, and CNS disease.

LABORATORY

The most common laboratory abnormalities seen are an elevation of the levels of muscle enzymes, greater than 90%, such as aspartate aminotransferase, lactate dehydrogenase, creatine kinase, and aldolase. Muscle enzymes may return to normal within a few months of disease onset if the child is treated adequately at times when disease remains active. The ESR may be normal in 30–50% of children. Up to 75% of children may also have a positive ANA, but the extractable nuclear antigens may be negative. The p155/140 kDa doublet protein has been found in 30% of children with JDM and may

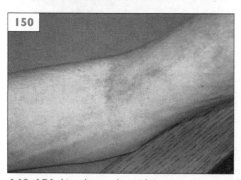

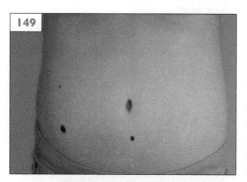

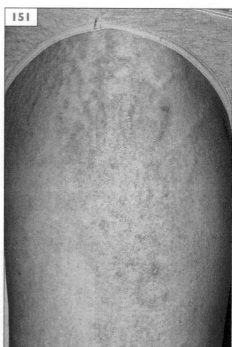

149–151 Lipodystrophy with increase in truncal fat (149); poikiloderma, a brown skin discoloration (150); striae and cutaneous erythema (151).

correlate with extensive cutaneous involvement. Finally, approximately 10% of children have myositis-specific antibodies and myositis-associated antibodies such as Jo-1, PL-7 (threonyl-tRNA synthetase), PL-12 (alanyl-tRNA synthetase), anti-signal recognition particle, and anti-MI-2, which define clinical subsets and predictors of disease severity. Autoantibodies to the tRNA synthetases have been associated with the clinical presentation of fever, inflammatory arthritis, interstitial lung disease, Raynaud phenomenon, and mechanic's hands.

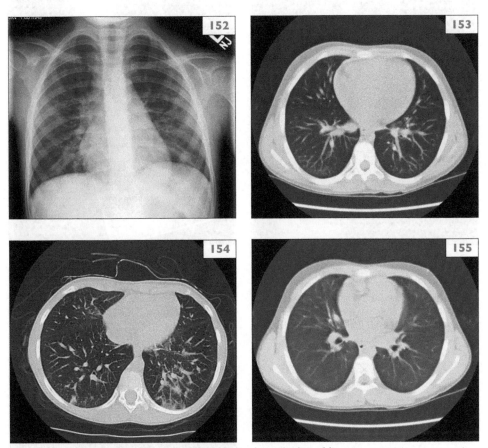

152–155 Interstitial lung disease in JDM including bronchiolitis obliterans organizing pneumonia (**152**); interstitial lung disease in JDM including ground-glass changes (**153, 154, 155**).

IMAGING

Plain radiography does not generally play a large role in the workup or therapeutic decision management of JDM. However, areas of calcinosis may be detected over the extremities or joints in plain radiographs (**156**) and cortical thickening of long bones can also be seen (**157**). MRI with T2-weighted fat suppression and STIR technique is useful in illustrating muscle edema, suggesting muscle inflammation (**158**). There may be cutaneous, subcutaneous, and fascial inflammation. MRI may help to localize an area for muscle biopsy. Finally, MRI may detect areas of calcinosis in JDM (**159**). Muscle ultrasound is generally not used in the diagnostic workup, but may reveal increased muscle echogenicity and attenuation. However, muscle ultrasound may be used to localize and monitor calcinosis (**160**).

DIFFERENTIAL DIAGNOSIS

Given the extensive skin findings seen in JDM, the diagnosis may initially be confused with SLE or scleroderma. Other connective tissue disease mimickers include juvenile idiopathic arthritis and juvenile polyarteritis nodosa.

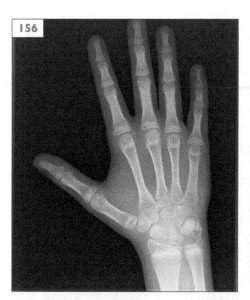

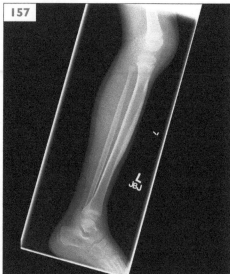

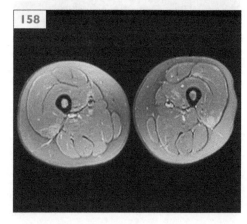

156–158 Radiograph of right hand showing soft tissue calcification around the third metacarpal head and the ulnar area in a child with JDM (**156**); cortical thickening of the tibia reported in a child with JDM (**157**); edema of the muscle in JDM (**158**).

Other childhood muscle diseases that resemble myositis include the muscular dystrophies, Duchenne and Becker, and the metabolic myopathies. Other disease entities to consider are sarcoid, viral myositis, celiac disease, and IBDs (*Table 22*).

PROGNOSIS

Prior to the use of corticosteroids, the prognosis of JDM was poor. Approximately one-third of children died from the disease and another third suffered from severe functional disability. With adequate and early treatment, however, children are now able to live normal lives. Calcinosis cutis has been a major cause of morbidity due to cosmetic disfigurement, contractures, and ulcerations resulting in secondary skin infections.

MANAGEMENT

A multidisciplinary approach involving consultations with a pediatric rheumatologist, dermatologist, and a physical and an occupational therapist are essential to reduce long-term morbidity. Assessment scales of strength and physical endurance such as the Childhood

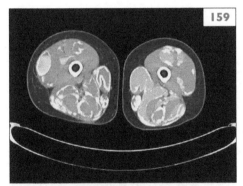

159 Cross-sectional CT scan of bilateral thighs demonstrating diffuse sheets of calcification along the myofascial planes of both thighs in JDM.

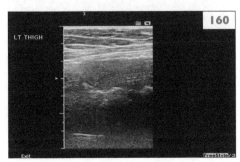

160 Ultrasound of liquid calcinosis.

| Table 22 |
Differential diagnosis of juvenile dermatomyositis
Connective tissue diseases
Systemic lupus erythematosus
Scleroderma
Mixed connective tissue disease
Juvenile idiopathic arthritis
Juvenile polyarteritis nodosa
ANCA + vasculitis
Muscular dystrophies
Duchenne
Becker
Metabolic myopathies
McArdle disease
Pompe disease
Other diseases
Sarcoid myopathy
Postinfectious myositis
Celiac disease
Inflammatory bowel disease
Myasthenia gravis
Leukemia
Multicentric reticulohistiocytosis

Health Assessment Questionnaire (CHAQ) and the Childhood Myositis Assessment Scale (CMAS) (*Table 23*) determine the clinical status and predict functional outcomes. Rehabilitation with physical therapy using isometric and isotonic exercises should be first-line management to restore and maintain muscle strength. To treat skin manifestations, sun avoidance and sunscreen that protects against UVA and UVB rays are important. Medical therapy for calcinosis has been controversial due to lack of adequate response; generally diltiazem or bisphosphonates have been used with varying success. Calcium and vitamin D supplementation is thought to be key in bone health.

For treatment of active muscle disease, oral corticosteroids are the backbone of therapy with high doses (1–2 mg/kg per day) initially used to induce remission over 4–6 weeks with a slow taper. Weaning of corticosteroids may take 2 years and when additional immunosuppressive agents are used weaning may at times occur over 1 year. For severe or refractory disease, pulse therapy with intravenous methylprednisolone of 30 mg/kg per day for 3 days should be used. Other immunosuppressive agents are added, at the onset of disease, to the corticosteroid regimen to reduce steroid side effects, disease relapse, and progressive disease. A commonly used agent is methotrexate with folic acid supplementation. Other immunosuppressive agents used include IVIG, cyclosporine, and rituximab. Combination therapy is often used as two agents generally work better to induce a rapid response and this is associated with less steroid toxicity.

COMPLICATIONS

Calcinosis cutis, interstitial lung disease, and GI involvement (including perforation) may occur in severe cases. Complications from long-term corticosteroid treatment may occur such as obesity, growth failure, acne, cataracts, hypertension, menstrual irregularities, psychiatric disturbances, avascular necrosis (**161**), osteoporosis, steroid myopathy, lipodystrophy, and metabolic toxicities such as insulin resistance and hypertriglyceridemia. Opportunistic infections can occur from corticosteroids and other immunosuppressive therapies used to treat JDM.

Table 23
Childhood Myositis Assessment Scale (details in Lovell *et al.* 1999)

1 Head elevation
2 Leg raise/touch object
3 Straight-leg lift
4 Supine to prone
5 Sit-ups
6 Supine to sit
7 Arm raise/straighten
8 Arm raise/duration
9 Floor sit
10 All-fours maneuver
11 Floor rise
12 Chair rise
13 Stool step
14 Pick up

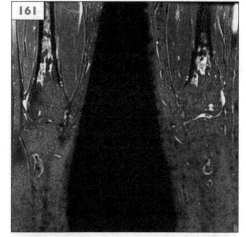

161 T2-weighted fat-saturated MR scan of a JDM patient on intravenous steroids with avascular necrosis of the femur and tibia.

Juvenile polymyositis

DEFINITION
Juvenile polymyositis (JPM) is less common than JDM. It is a systemic autoimmune disease of the muscles without skin involvement. Diagnosis is based on the Bohan and Peter criteria which involve proximal muscle weakness, elevated muscle enzymes, myopathic findings on EMG, and muscle biopsy with inflammation.

EPIDEMIOLOGY AND ETIOLOGY
JPM is an extremely rare childhood myopathy. Because of its rarity, the incidence of JPM is unknown. As in JDM, girls are affected more than boys with a sex ratio of 2–5:1. The age of onset of JPM is similar to JDM with the highest incidence occurring in ages 5–10 years.

The etiology of JPM is largely unknown. As in JDM, similar environmental triggers and genetic risk factors have been associated with JPM. Infectious agents implicated in the development of JPM include viral such as Coxsackie B and respiratory syncytial virus, and bacterial infections such as *Streptococcus* spp. Non-infectious associations include drugs such as penicillamine, vaccines such as hepatitis B and BCG, as well as after bone marrow transplantations as in a graft-versus-host disease paradigm.

Pathogenesis of JPM likely involves the innate and adaptive immune system including the cell-mediated pathways causing muscle damage. Cytotoxic CD8+ T cells infiltrate muscle fibers and there is endomysial inflammation.

CLINICAL HISTORY
Children with JPM do not have the characteristic skin rash as seen in JDM. Muscle weakness is the hallmark feature, usually occurring in the deltoids and the quadriceps muscles; sometimes it is severe resulting in hypotonia. Similar to JDM, constitutional symptoms may occur prior to obvious muscle weakness. The child may have difficulty getting out of bed or tire easily in physical education classes or sporting events. A non-erosive arthritis, dysphonia, hoarseness, esophageal dysmotility, and muscle pain are other associated features.

PHYSICAL EXAMINATION
Symmetric, proximal muscle weakness is seen in all children, although distal muscles may be affected as well. Muscle involvement usually occurs in the deltoids and the quadriceps muscles, or both muscle groups. There are no cutaneous or nailfold capillary abnormalities. As with JDM, the child may demonstrate an abnormal Gower maneuver with an inability to rise to a standing position without the use of the arms.

LABORATORY
The most common laboratory abnormalities are an elevation in the levels of muscle enzymes such as aspartate aminotransferase, lactate dehydrogenase, creatine kinase, and aldolase. Muscle enzymes may return to normal within a few months of disease onset if the child is treated adequately.

Similar myositis-associated and myositis-specific autoantibodies have been seen in JPM as in JDM. These autoantibodies include Jo-1, PL-7 (threonyl-tRNA synthetase), PL-12 (alanyl-tRNA synthetase), anti-signal recognition particle, and anti-MI-2, which define clinical subsets and predictors of disease severity. Autoantibodies to the tRNA synthetases have been associated with the clinical presentation of fever, inflammatory arthritis, interstitial lung disease, Raynaud phenomenon, and mechanic's hands. Autoantibodies to the signal recognition particle have been observed in African–American girls with more aggressive and refractory disease, or cardiac manifestations.

IMAGING
Plain films do not play a large role in the workup or management of JPM. As in JDM, MRI with T2-weighted fat suppression and STIR technique is useful in illustrating muscle edema, suggesting muscle inflammation, and the signal intensity from STIR may correlate with the level of disease activity. With chronic muscle disease, there may be fatty infiltration of the muscle and/or muscle atrophy. As in JDM, muscle ultrasound generally is not used in the diagnostic workup, but may reveal increased muscle echogenicity and attenuation.

DIFFERENTIAL DIAGNOSIS
As with JDM, the childhood muscle diseases that mimic myositis include the muscular dystrophies, Duchenne and Becker, and the metabolic myopathies. Evaluation with muscle biopsy is key to differentiate JPM from other causes of myopathy.

PROGNOSIS

The course may be protracted and refractory to steroids. Complications from steroid treatment such as obesity, growth failure, acne, cataracts, hypertension, menstrual irregularities, psychiatric disturbances, avascular necrosis, osteoporosis, steroid myopathy, lipodystrophy, and metabolic toxicities may occur.

MANAGEMENT

As in JDM, a multidisciplinary approach involving a pediatric rheumatologist and a physical and occupational therapist is needed to reduce long-term morbidity. Assessment scales of strength and physical endurance such as the CHAQ and the CMAS have been developed to determine and predict functional outcomes. Rehabilitation with isometric and isotonic exercises should be the first-line management of childhood myositis to restore and maintain muscle strength.

For treatment of active muscle disease, oral corticosteroids are the backbone of therapy with high doses (1–2 mg/kg per day) initially used to induce remission over 4–6 weeks with a slow taper to avoid relapse. However, JPM is often chronic and may be refractory to steroids. Weaning of corticosteroids may take 2 years or longer. For severe or refractory disease, it is recommended to use pulse therapy with intravenous methylprednisolone of 30 mg/kg per day for 3 days. Other immunosuppressive agents are added to reduce steroid side effects, disease relapse, and progressive disease. As in JDM, a commonly used immunosuppressant is methotrexate with folic acid supplementation. Other immunosuppressive agents used include IVIG, cyclosporine, anti-TNF agents such as etanercept and infliximab, and rituximab. Combination therapy is often used in the treatment of childhood myositis as two agents together generally work better to induce a rapid response.

COMPLICATIONS

Muscle atrophy and interstitial lung disease may occur in severe cases. Complications from long-term corticosteroid treatment may occur such as obesity, growth failure, acne, cataracts, hypertension, menstrual irregularities, psychiatric disturbances, avascular necrosis (see **161**), osteoporosis, steroid myopathy, lipodystrophy, and metabolic toxicities such as insulin resistance and hypertriglyceridemia. Opportunistic infections can occur from corticosteroids and other immunuosuppressive therapies used to treat JDM.

Postinfectious myositis

DEFINITION
Postinfectious myositis is a transient myositis following an acute infection.

EPIDEMIOLOGY AND ETIOLOGY
Children and adolescents are affected, usually boys more than girls. Viruses associated with myositis include influenza A and B and Coxsackie B viruses. Other infectious causes include toxoplasmosis, *Trichinella spiralis*, and staphylococcal and streptococcal bacteremia. Also, clostridia, *Salmonella* spp., and schistosomiasis are less common causes. Pyomyositis, as from *Staphylococcus* spp., is a skeletal muscle abscess occurring after a local injury.

CLINICAL HISTORY
Coxsackie B virus may cause a pleurodynia with chest wall pain and fever after a headache, nausea, vomiting, and sore throat. Illness lasts 3–5 days. Trichinosis may cause fever, diarrhea, and abdominal pain. Pyomyositis may be associated with a low-grade fever.

PHYSICAL EXAMINATION
Focal tenderness of involved muscles such as the thigh, buttock, and calf muscles is present. Trichinosis may cause periorbital edema and facial swelling. If pyomyositis is present, the affected muscle may be warm and tender.

LABORATORY
Elevated serum muscle enzymes are usually seen such as creatine kinase and aspartate aminotransferase. Myositis associated with schistosomiasis or trichinosis may be associated with marked peripheral blood eosinophilia.

IMAGING
Ultrasound may localize the muscle abscess with pyomyositis.

DIFFERENTIAL DIAGNOSIS
As with JDM and JPM, the childhood muscle diseases that mimic myositis include the muscular dystrophies and the metabolic myopathies. Postinfectious myopathies would more often be seen in the acute setting, associated with the above-mentioned infectious symptoms.

PROGNOSIS
The illness should be self-limited. Proper treatment of the bacterial, parasite, or fungal infection should result in prompt recovery.

MANAGEMENT
Postinfectious myositis is usually self-limited, but glucocorticoids may be used to treat the inflammation. Mebendazole or thiabendazole is used to treat trichinosis.

COMPLICATIONS
There are usually no long-term complications from the muscle involvement.

CHAPTER 6

Vasculitis

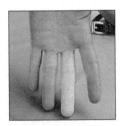
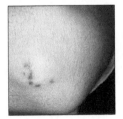
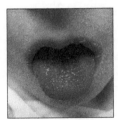
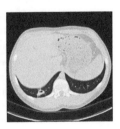

Vasculitis involves inflammation of blood vessels. Beyond this straightforward description, however, lies a family of complex and protean disorders. As a result of the ubiquity of blood vessels, the variability of their structure and function, and the multitude of ways in which they may be affected, vasculitis can lead to anything from numbness to pain, thrombosis to bleeding, aneurysms to obstruction.

Large gaps in the understanding of nosology, etiology, and pathogenesis confound the study of vasculitis. This lack of information, in turn, complicates attempts at classification. Primary vasculitides may be classified according to their clinical manifestations, the size of blood vessels involved, the histology of vascular damage, or the presumed disease pathogenesis. This chapter uses a working scheme for classifying pediatric vasculitides, attempting to include current knowledge of disease pathogenesis but leaving open the possibility of reclassification as new data emerge (*Table 24*).

Table 24
Childhood vasculitides

Large-vessel diseases
　Takayasu arteritis
　Giant cell (temporal) arteritis

Medium-vessel disease
　Polyarteritis nodosa
　Cutaneous
　Systemic
　Cogan syndrome
　Kawasaki disease

Small-vessel disease
　Henoch–Schönlein purpura
　Hypersensitivity vasculitis
　Primary angiitis of the central nervous system
　ANCA-positive vasculitis
　Wegener granulomatosis
　Microscopic periarteritis
　Churg–Strauss syndrome

Kawasaki disease

DEFINITION
Kawasaki disease (KD), or mucocutaneous lymph node syndrome, is unusual among the vasculitides in being a self-limited condition, with fever and manifestations of acute inflammation lasting for an average of 12 days without therapy. It is diagnosed by clinical criteria, not histology or angiography.

EPIDEMIOLOGY AND ETIOLOGY
KD is almost entirely a disease of children. The average age of patients with KD is about 2 years, 80–90% of cases occur before the fifth birthday, and occurrence beyond late childhood is extremely rare. Boys are affected 50% more frequently than girls. Asians are affected 5–10 times as frequently as whites; blacks and Hispanics have an intermediate risk.

The etiology of KD is unclear, but vascular damage likely plays a role. Blood vessel damage in KD results from an aberrant immune response leading to endothelial cell injury and vessel wall damage. Genetic factors seem to account for the varying susceptibility of different ethnic groups to KD, with polymorphisms of chemokines and TNF receptors and variations in HLA haplotypes all possibly contributing. After many failed attempts to find a single etiologic agent, many researchers now believe that KD represents a final common pathway of immune-mediated vascular inflammation following a variety of inciting infections.

The fever and systemic inflammation of KD reflect elevated levels of proinflammatory cytokines such as TNF, IL-1, and IL-6 that are also thought to mediate the underlying vascular inflammation. Pathologically, the finding of macrophages and IgA-producing plasma cells in vessel walls of children with KD is unique.

CLINICAL HISTORY
Guidelines for the diagnosis of KD were established by Tomisaku Kawasaki in 1967 (*Table 25*). The diagnosis requires the presence of fever lasting 5 days or more without any other explanation, combined with at least four of five manifestations of mucocutaneous inflammation. Children who do not meet the criteria may none-the-less develop coronary artery changes. In an attempt to identify patients with this incomplete form of KD, an

AHA working group has recommended modifications of the criteria.

PHYSICAL EXAMINATION

Fever in KD is above 38.5°C and typically hectic and minimally responsive to antipyretic agents. Bilateral non-exudative bulbar conjunctivitis is present in as many as 90% of cases of KD. Children are also frequently photophobic, and many develop anterior uveitis. Mucositis, marked by cracked, red lips and a strawberry tongue (162), is characteristic; discrete oral lesions, such as vesicles or ulcers, as well as tonsillar exudate, suggest a viral or bacterial infection rather than KD. Cutaneous manifestations of KD are polymorphous. The rash typically begins as perineal erythema and desquamation, followed by macular, morbilliform, or targetoid lesions of the trunk and extremities. Vesicular or bullous lesions are rare. Late in the course of the disease, children develop extremity changes, including indurated edema of the dorsum of the hands and feet and diffuse erythema of the palms and soles. The convalescent phase of KD may be characterized by sheet-like desquamation that begins in the periungual region of the hands and feet (163) and by linear nail creases (Beau's lines). In addition, one-third of children have a self-limited small-joint polyarthritis during the first week of illness. Cervical lymphadenopathy is the least consistent of the cardinal features of KD, absent in as many as 50% of children with the disease. When present, lymphadenopathy tends to involve primarily the anterior cervical nodes overlying the sternocleidomastoid muscle, while diffuse lymphadenopathy or splenomegaly should prompt a search for alternative diagnoses.

LABORATORY

Systemic inflammation manifested by elevation of acute-phase reactants (e.g. CRP, ESR, and α_1-antitrypsin), leukocytosis, and a left shift in the WBC count is characteristic. By the second week of illness, platelet counts may reach $1,000,000/mm^3$ in the most severe cases.

Table 25
Criteria for diagnosis of Kawasaki disease (numbers in parentheses indicate the approximate percentage of children with Kawasaki disease who display the criterion) (modified from Centers for Disease Control 1990)

Fever >5 days, not explained by another disease process (4 days if treatment with IVIG eradicates fever), plus at least four of the following clinical signs:

- Bilateral conjunctival injection (80–90%)
- Changes in the oropharyngeal mucous membranes (including one or more of: injected and/or fissured lips, strawberry tongue, injected pharynx) (80–90%)
- Changes in the peripheral extremities, including erythema and/or edema of the hands and feet (acute phase) or periungual desquamation (convalescent phase) (80%)
- Polymorphous rash, primarily truncal; non-vesicular (>90%)
- Cervical lymphadenopathy with at least one node >1.5 cm (50–75%)

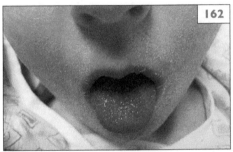

162 Strawberry tongue in Kawasaki disease.

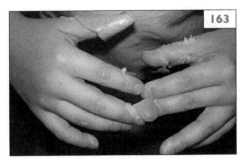

163 Sheet-like desquamation in Kawasaki disease.

Children with KD often present with a normocytic, normochromic anemia, and urinalysis commonly reveals microscopic pyuria. Intrahepatic congestion often leads to elevated transaminase levels or mild hyperbilirubinemia. CSF typically displays a mononuclear pleocytosis with normal sugar and protein, and arthrocentesis of involved joints demonstrates 50,000–300,000 white cells/mm^3, primarily neutrophils.

IMAGING

An echocardiogram should be obtained early in the acute phase of illness; up to 20–25% of children develop coronary artery aneurysms within 10 days of the onset of fever if not treated with IVIG. Abdominal ultrasound often shows hydrops of the gallbladder, especially in children with fullness and tenderness of the right upper quadrant. Coronary angiography is rarely necessary as echocardiograms adequately visualize involved vessels in most children.

DIFFERENTIAL DIAGNOSIS

KD is most commonly confused with infectious exanthems of childhood. Measles, echovirus, and adenovirus may share many of the signs of mucocutaneous inflammation, but they typically cause less inflammation and lack the extremity changes seen in KD. Toxin-mediated illnesses, especially β-hemolytic streptococcal infection and toxic shock syndrome, lack the ocular and articular involvement typical of KD. Drug reactions such as Stevens–Johnson syndrome or serum sickness may mimic KD but with subtle differences in the ocular and mucosal manifestations. Systemic-onset JRA is marked by prominent rash, fever, and systemic inflammation, and may be difficult to distinguish from KD until persistent polyarthritis becomes evident.

PROGNOSIS

Although most small aneurysms fully resolve by echocardiogram, there is a concern that vascular reactivity may not return to normal despite grossly normal appearance. Children should thus be followed indefinitely after KD, and additional cardiac risk factors should be monitored closely. Overall, with modern treatment and follow-up, the prognosis of children with KD is excellent: 25-year follow-up of Japanese children without persistent coronary artery abnormalities demonstrates no increase in morbidity or mortality.

MANAGEMENT

Patients who fulfill the criteria for KD are hospitalized and treated with IVIG and aspirin. IVIG therapy within the first 10 days of illness reduces the incidence of coronary artery aneurysms by more than 70%. Fever persists or returns within 48 hours after treatment in 10–15% of patients. These children are at increased risk of developing coronary artery aneurysms, so they are treated with an additional dose of IVIG, one to three daily doses of pulsed methylprednisolone (30 mg/kg), or a single dose of infliximab (5 mg/kg). When symptoms are prolonged beyond 3–4 weeks, consideration should be given to an alternative diagnosis, including chronic vasculitides such as polyarteritis nodosa (PAN).

Patients suspected of having KD but not meeting diagnostic criteria may require further testing such as slit-lamp examination and echocardiography to confirm the diagnosis. At times, children are treated for suspected KD when the diagnosis is uncertain but no clear alternative explanation for the clinical findings can be identified. Markers of increased risk of developing coronary artery aneurysms, including age under 1 year, severe systemic inflammation, or consumptive coagulopathy, may shift the balance toward empiric therapy.

COMPLICATIONS

The primary complication is the development of coronary artery disease as noted above. Rarely other cardiac involvement occurs, such as myocarditis. Complications of therapy include risk of bleeding with aspirin and hypersensitivity to IVIG.

Henoch–Schönlein pupura

DEFINITION

Henoch–Schönlein purpura (HSP) is a small-vessel leukocytoclastic vasculitis that presents as the triad of non-thrombocytopenic palpable purpura, arthritis, and colicky abdominal pain. HSP is diagnosed on the basis of clinical findings; vascular imaging and biopsy are generally neither necessary nor diagnostic.

EPIDEMIOLOGY AND ETIOLOGY

HSP is the most common vasculitis in children, occurring in up to 1 child in 5,000 per year. Similar to Kawasaki disease, most cases occur in children under 7 years of age, almost twice as many boys as girls contract the condition, and peak incidence tends to be during the colder winter months.

HSP appears to represent an aberrant immune response to an infectious or antigenic stimulus. Infections, especially upper respiratory tract infections (most commonly streptococcal), precede the onset of illness in at least 50% of children with HSP, but immunizations and insect bites may also trigger the condition. As yet unidentified host and pathogen factors determine a child's likelihood of developing this vasculitis.

In HSP, the alternate pathway of complement activated by large IgA-containing immune complexes may be important, though precisely how this contributes to the HSP phenotype is poorly understood. Small vessels have a perivascular infiltrate consisting of neutrophils and mononuclear cells, and deposits of IgA, C3, and fibrin may be detected using immunofluorescence and electron microscopy. Renal biopsies typically show an endocapillary proliferative glomerulonephritis involving endothelial and mesangial cells. Proliferation of extracapillary cells also may occur, resulting in variable degrees of crescent formation.

CLINICAL HISTORY

Skin involvement in HSP may begin as urticaria; in most cases it progresses to palpable purpuric lesions primarily involving dependent areas (buttocks and lower legs in ambulatory children, the sacrum, ears and buttocks in infants) (**164**). Arthritis may affect any joint in an asymmetric and migratory pattern, though lower extremities are more commonly involved. GI involvement ranges from colicky abdominal pain to profuse bleeding, intussusception, and perforation. Renal disease usually is observed more than 10 days after the onset of illness.

PHYSICAL EXAMINATION

Children often appear well and are afebrile despite having prominent purpura. Edema may involve the scrotum (**165**), dorsa of the hands or feet, and even the scalp. The arthritis of HSP is transient, causing neither chronic joint changes nor permanent sequelae. Signs of the syndrome recur within 6 weeks in up to 40% of children, most commonly abdominal pain and rash. Exacerbations are usually shorter in duration and the symptoms are generally milder than those of the initial disease.

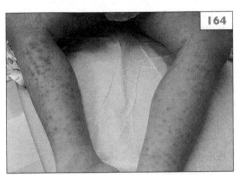

164 Lower extremity purpuric rash in HSP.

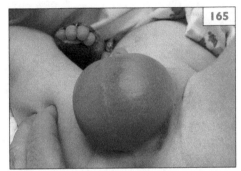

165 Severe scrotal edema in HSP.

LABORATORY

HSP is a clinical diagnosis; no specific laboratory abnormalities are characteristic. Laboratory tests usually reflect the triggering infection rather than the HSP itself, so investigations are generally limited to ruling out other vasculitides, infections, and hematologic disorders. Children should have a CBC to exclude thrombocytopenia as a cause of palpable purpura, and in some cases measurement of PT, aPTT, and D-dimers to rule out coagulopathies. BUN and creatinine levels and urinalysis are monitored to evaluate renal involvement. In severe cases, renal biopsy is helpful for excluding other causes of acute nephritis, nephrotic syndrome, or renal failure, and for estimating prognosis.

IMAGING

Imaging is generally limited to assessing the cause of abdominal pain in children with known or suspected HSP. Plain radiographs reveal free air in cases of ruptured viscus, and abdominal ultrasound is the examination of choice for determining whether an ileo-ileal intussusception has occurred. Since primarily small vessels are involved, skin or renal biopsies are generally more helpful than vascular imaging if definitive evidence of vasculitis is needed.

DIFFERENTIAL DIAGNOSIS

Clinicians must consider infectious and noninfectious causes of purpura. Sepsis, malignant, and metabolic causes of disseminated intravascular coagulopathy or thrombocytopenia can generally be excluded clinically, based on the relatively slow tempo of disease progression and well appearance of the patient. Exclusion of other vasculitides causing palpable purpura, especially hypersensitivity vasculitis, Wegener granulomatosis, and Churg–Strauss syndrome, might require testing for ANCA, serum complement levels, or even a skin biopsy. Acute hemorrhagic edema of infancy (**166**), a benign febrile condition of infants, presents with ecchymotic-like macular purpura distinct from that of HSP.

PROGNOSIS

HSP is a self-limited illness that typically resolves within a month in two-thirds of children. Younger patients tend to have milder disease of shorter duration, while adults have a higher incidence of severe renal involvement. Generally there is a correlation between the severity of urinary abnormalities and the chances of developing chronic renal disease, with those demonstrating both nephritic and nephrotic changes at greatest risk. Overall about 1–5% of patients with HSP develop some degree of chronic renal disease.

MANAGEMENT

Therapy of HSP is primarily supportive, aiming for symptomatic relief of arthritis and abdominal pain. Acetaminophen or NSAIDs appear to be effective and safe in most cases. Use of steroids, whether in children who fail to respond to NSAIDs or in those thought to be at highest risk of developing renal compromise, is controversial. Prednisone at a dose of 1–2 mg/kg per day appears to rapidly relieve symptoms in the majority of cases, but caregivers must avoid excessively rapid tapering of the steroids, as this commonly triggers a flare of symptoms. More potent immunosuppressive agents are reserved for children with biopsy-proven crescentic glomerulonephritis or other life-threatening complications such as cerebral or pulmonary hemorrhage.

COMPLICATIONS

Renal insufficinecy can occasionally occur. Rarely, intestinal perforation has been reported. Potential complications related to therapy include gastritis with NSAIDs and opportunistic infection with corticosteroids.

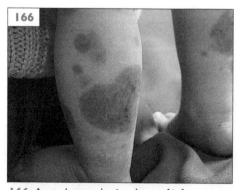

166 Acute hemorrhagic edema of infancy.

Polyarteritis nodosa

DEFINITION

Polyarteritis nodosa (PAN) is a systemic necrotizing vasculitis affecting medium and/or small arteries. The segmental panmural fibrinoid necrosis with nodule and aneurysm formation give this condition its name. PAN is important historically as the first non-infectious cause of vascular damage to be identified, but at least one-third of children have a more limited cutaneous form that is restricted largely to the skin and joints. Diagnosis of PAN usually requires tissue biopsy and/or radiological documentation of vasculitis.

EPIDEMIOLOGY AND ETIOLOGY

Worldwide, PAN is most commonly associated with hepatitis B or C infections. Perhaps as a result of the relative infrequency of these infections in children, pediatric PAN is quite rare, especially in North America. Childhood incidence of PAN peaks at 9–10 years of age, and it may be slightly more common in boys than in girls.

PAN is characterized by transmural necrosis of the walls of medium-sized arteries. Both the patchy, interrupted involvement and the association with hepatitis B suggest an immune-complex-mediated process. The resulting recruitment of polymorphonuclear neutrophils and monocytes, leading to focal areas of necrosis, is typical of an Arthus reaction.

The prevalence of systemic PAN in adults with chronic hepatitis suggests that the development of vasculitis is related to the disordered formation or clearance of immune complexes. Although no clear genetic association has been identified, the fact that up to 1% of patients with familial Mediterranean fever (FMF) develop PAN raises the possibility that inflammasomes play a role.

CLINICAL HISTORY

Cutaneous PAN is usually limited to the skin and musculoskeletal system. It commonly occurs after a sore throat or streptococcal pharyngitis. Livedo reticularis, maculopapular rash, painful skin nodules, edema, and arthritis mostly affect the knees and ankles. Constitutional symptoms are generally mild and systemic involvement is, by definition, rare. Symptoms are more troubling than disabling,

and treatment generally consists of NSAIDs and steroids.

Systemic PAN may involve virtually any muscular artery. Consequently, in addition to constitutional symptoms, it may cause a vast array of organ dysfunction. Palpable purpura, livedo, acral blanching (**167**), necrotic dermal lesions and autoamputation (**168**), abdominal pain, arthritis/arthralgia, myositis/myalgia, renovascular hypertension, neurologic deficits, pulmonary disease, and coronary arteritis may all be seen at presentation or during the course of the disease.

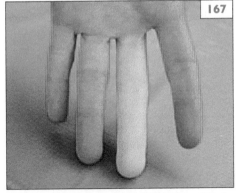

167 Acral blanching due to PAN of the digital artery.

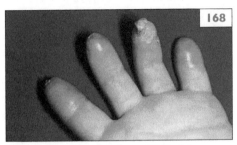

168 Autoamputation due to PAN of the fingers.

PHYSICAL EXAMINATION

Evidence of cutaneous PAN is generally limited to rashes such as livedo reticularis or nodules ('nodosa') overlying medium-sized vessels. Arthritis and fever frequently accompany these findings, but other organ systems are rarely involved. Systemic PAN, on the other hand, may involve any organ system, so evidence of this protean and widespread condition may lead to anything from cranial nerve palsies and myocardial infarction to testicular pain and an acute abdomen.

LABORATORY

Laboratory evaluation usually reflects the ongoing systemic inflammation including anemia, leukocytosis, thrombocytosis, and elevated ESR, CRP, and immunoglobulins. Evidence of myositis (elevated creatine kinase and aldolase) and renal dysfunction (increased BUN and creatinine) are also common findings. Complement levels are normal.

IMAGING

Vessels affected by PAN typically demonstrate the so-called 'beading' of arteries, representing alternating narrowing and dilation of high-pressure vessels. CT or MR angiography is generally preferred to conventional angiography because they are less invasive and have less potential for complications (169a–c). Echocardiography may be used to visualize coronary arteries when cardiac involvement is suspected. None-the-less, in some patients, conventional angiography may be necessary to determine the extent and severity of vascular involvement (170).

DIFFERENTIAL DIAGNOSIS

PAN should be considered in the differential diagnosis of any undiagnosed systemic inflammatory condition or in cases of severe, unexplained hypertension. As a result of its pleomorphism, PAN may be confused with other rheumatologic conditions including systemic-onset JRA, Kawasaki disease, and dermatomyositis. Appendicitis or hypercoagulability must be excluded when abdominal pain or vascular insufficiency is the presenting feature, and testicular torsion is a potential confounder when scrotal vessels are involved. Small vessels are spared in classic PAN, so glomerulonephritis typically is not a feature of this condition.

PROGNOSIS

Recent reviews of PAN in children suggest an excellent overall prognosis, with a 4-year mortality rate under 5%. Such an outcome is predicated, however, on close follow-up and aggressive management of active disease or its complications.

MANAGEMENT

In cutaneous PAN, treatment is primarily aimed at controlling symptoms. In systemic disease, on the other hand, vascular inflammation must be controlled in order to prevent compromise of vital vascular beds. In both cases the mainstay of therapy is high-dose steroids, but, since the disease tends to persist or relapse, many patients require steroid-sparing agents for long-term management. These may include methotrexate, IVIG, or TNF inhibitors. Penicillin prophylaxis may prevent disease flares due to recurrent streptococcal infections.

COMPLICATIONS

Renal insufficiency can occasionally occur. Organ ischemia may occur secondary to vascular damage. Potential complications related to therapy include gastritis with NSAIDs, avascular necrosis, and opportunistic infection with corticosteroids. Immunosuppressive medications are also associated with an increased risk of opportunistic infections.

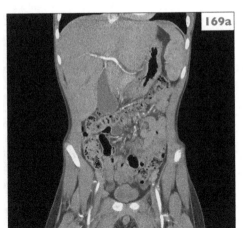

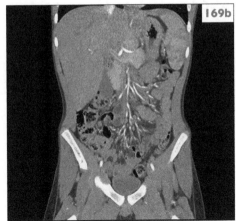

169a–c CT angiography showing hepatic artery narrowing (courtesy of Ann M. Reed, MD, Mayo Clinic) (**169a**); CT enterography showing mesenteric narrowing (courtesy of Ann M. Reed, MD, Mayo Clinic) (**169b**); CT enterography showing renal infarcts (courtesy of Ann M. Reed, MD, Mayo Clinic) (**169c**).

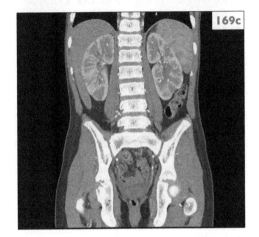

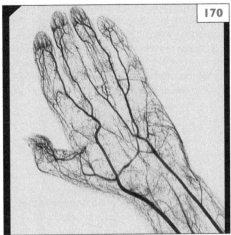

170 Obstruction of the fourth digital artery in PAN.

ANCA-associated vasculitides

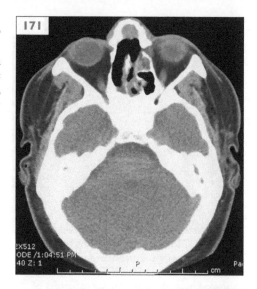

DEFINITION
ANCA-associated vasculitides (AAVs) are a group of conditions marked by pauci-immune inflammation of the vessels of the lungs, kidneys, and skin in the presence of anti-neutrophil cytoplasmic antibodies. They include:

- Churg–Strauss syndrome (CSS) – a cause of steroid-dependent asthma with pulmonary infiltrates and systemic inflammation accompanied by ANCA in either a cytoplasmic or a peripheral pattern.
- Wegener granulomatosis (WG) – a necrotizing granulomatous inflammation of small- to medium-sized vessels positive for cytoplasmic staining (c-ANCA) against the neutrophil protease PR-3.
- Microscopic polyangiitis (MPA) – a non-granulomatous necrotizing vasculitis of small vessels characterized by a positive p-ANCA with reactivity to MPO.

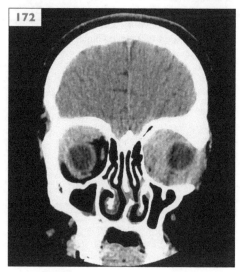

EPIDEMIOLOGY AND ETIOLOGY
The total incidence of pediatric AAVs appears to be on the order of one new case per million children per year. The first report of CSS occurring in a pre-teen has been published only in the past decade, so, while these conditions must be included in the differential diagnosis of inflammatory disorders of the kidneys and lungs, most practitioners will not see a case during their careers.

These conditions share antibodies to antigens within the neutrophil cytoplasm and a microscopic pauci-immune polyangiitis marked by little or no complement deposition. They primarily target the respiratory, renal, and cutaneous systems, and they often develop in the wake of a viral infection. The genetic and environmental factors responsible for their development, however, are not known.

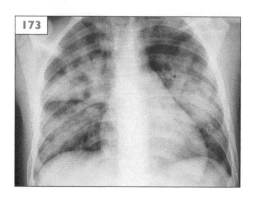

171–173 Sinus CT in Wegener granulomatosus (**171**); pseudotumor of the orbit in a PR-3+ child (courtesy of Ann M. Reed, MD, Mayo Clinic) (**172**); pulmonary hemorrhage in Wegener granulomatosus (**173**).

The pathogenesis of AAVs appears to be related to ANCA. These antibodies most likely stabilize adherence of rolling neutrophils to endothelium, and activate neutrophils and monocytes to undergo an oxidative burst. Activation of phagocytic cells causes upregulation of proinflammatory cytokines (such as TNF-α and IL-8), with resultant localized endothelial cell cytotoxicity.

CLINICAL HISTORY

Clinical manifestations of AAVs in children are similar to those in adults. Children with WG almost universally have nasal and sinus involvement and respiratory disease including pulmonary hemorrhage (**171–173**).

Arthralgias, ocular findings, and skin (**174**) or renal involvement (**175**) occur in more than half, while GI disease and CNS involvement are less typical. Unique to pediatric series is a high frequency of subglottic stenosis, noted in almost 50% of children with WG (**176**). CSS presents initially as allergic rhinitis and asthma. After months or years, peripheral eosinophilia and pulmonary infiltrates develop (**177**). Only later do manifestations of systemic vasculitis become evident, with weight loss, fever, arthralgia, myalgia, nodular rash, and neuropathy. MPA is most commonly limited to the kidneys, though the presence of constitutional and inflammatory involvement demonstrate the systemic nature of the condition.

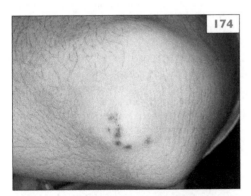

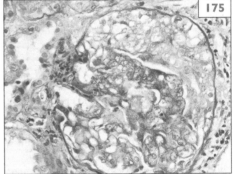

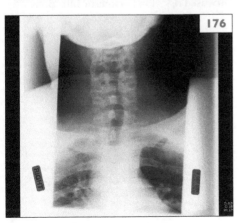

174–175 Cutaneous vasculitis in Wegener granulomatosus (courtesy of Ann M. Reed, MD, Mayo Clinic) (**174**); crescent formation and glomerular collapse due to Wegener granulomatosus (courtesy of Michael Somers, MD) (**175**); glottic and subglottic stenosis in Wegener granulomatosus (**176**).

PHYSICAL EXAMINATION

Most children with WG present with upper respiratory symptoms such as epistaxis, sinusitis, otitis media, or hearing loss, or with cough, wheezing, or dyspnea indicative of lower respiratory tract involvement. Similarly, children with CSS are recognized to have asthma, but then their symptoms worsen and become increasingly refractory to routine management. Unusually persistent or severe manifestations, or development of hemoptysis or hypertension, suggest evolution beyond routine childhood illnesses.

LABORATORY

While specific ANCA targeted against PR-3 or MPO is positive in the majority of patients with AAVs, this autoantibody may also be found in other more common diseases such as cystic fibrosis and IBD. Accordingly, a positive ANCA should not replace a tissue biopsy in confirming the diagnosis of vasculitis, nor should ANCA screening substitute for a careful history and physical examination. Similarly, while peripheral eosinophilia is characteristic of active CSS, it is more frequently encountered in common allergic conditions, and therefore should be only one of many factors weighed during the diagnostic process.

IMAGING

Chest radiographs may be particularly helpful when a diagnosis of WG or CSS is suspected. Even in asymptomatic children with WG, up to one-third have radiographic abnormalities (**173, 178, 179**). Similarly, the majority of children with CSS demonstrate pulmonary infiltrates that would be atypical for uncomplicated asthma (**180**).

DIFFERENTIAL DIAGNOSIS

Biopsy or radiographic confirmation of vascular inflammation is necessary in order to confirm the diagnosis of AAVs, and to exclude a variety of other conditions that may have a non-specific ANCA. Necrotizing granulomatous vascular inflammation in a child with suggestive clinical features is strongly suggestive of WG. In CSS, biopsy of involved tissue shows significant perivascular eosinophilic infiltrates and occasional extravascular granulomas.

PROGNOSIS

Despite progress in the management of WG, the disease continues to cause significant morbidity and mortality due to relapses and treatment-related toxicity. Subglottic stenosis does not respond to systemic therapy, but rather requires surgical dilation and local steroid injections. In patients with limited upper respiratory disease trimethoprim/sulfamethoxazole has been shown to be beneficial, perhaps by suppressing URIs that might activate vascular inflammation.

MANAGEMENT

AAVs, especially WG, are rapidly progressive and may be fatal without effective immunosuppressive therapy. Consequently, potent combination therapies are the mainstay of therapy, including steroids, cyclophosphamide, azathioprine, methotrexate, and more recently mycophenolate mofetil and anti-TNF antibodies (but not the TNF-receptor antagonist etanercept). Most recently, rituximab has been proposed as a potential replacement for both cyclophosphamide and long-term steroids in AAVs.

COMPLICATIONS

Renal insufficiency can occasionally occur. Large airway disease may lead to subglottic stenosis. Organ ischemia may occur secondary to vascular damage. Nasal septal perforation has been reported. Potential complications related to therapy include gastritis with NSAIDs, avascular necrosis, and opportunistic infection with corticosteroids. Immunosuppressive medications are also associated with increased risk of opportunistic infections.

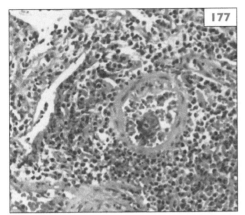

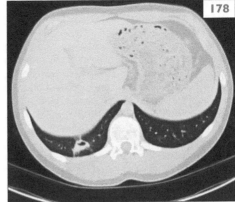

177–179 Eosinophilic pulmonary vasculitis in Churg–Strauss syndrome (courtesy of Sarah Vargas, MD and Debra Boyer, MD) (177); Wegener granulomatosus cavitary lesion (courtesy of Ann M. Reed, MD, Mayo Clinic) (178); Wegener granulomatosus cavitary lesion (courtesy of Ann M. Reed, MD, Mayo Clinic) (179).

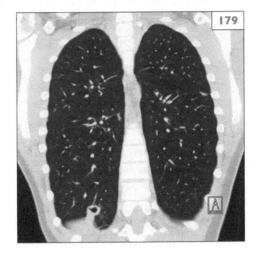

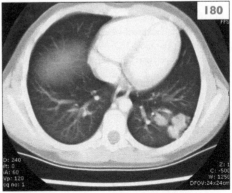

180 Chest CT scan in Churg–Strauss syndrome.

Takayasu arteritis

DEFINITION

Takayasu arteritis (TA), or 'pulseless disease,' is a large-vessel vasculitis that involves the aorta and its major branches. Although reports of patients losing their peripheral pulses have appeared for hundreds of years, TA is named after a Japanese ophthalmologist who first described, in 1908, the changes in retinal vessels due to increased outflow into unobstructed cerebral vessels.

EPIDEMIOLOGY AND ETIOLOGY

TA is the third most common form of childhood vasculitis. It most commonly develops during the third decade of life, but the disease has been reported in infancy. TA is more common in the Far East and West Africa than in Europe and North America. In a recent review of childhood TA the mean age of onset was 11.4 years and two-thirds of patients were female.

The cause of TA remains unknown, though histopathology and immunohistochemistry of biopsy and autopsy samples from adults with TA suggest a primarily T-cell-mediated mechanism. Certain HLA associations have been found in Japan, but these have not been confirmed in other populations.

TA lesions consist of granulomatous changes progressing from the vascular adventitia to the media, indistinguishable from those seen in giant cell and temporal arteritis. This histopathology, and the correlations between levels of IL-6 and RANTES and disease activity, suggest that T cells and macrophages play a central role in the disease.

CLINICAL HISTORY

TA is diagnosed on the basis of the distribution of involvement – primarily the aorta and its branches – and the young age of patients – typically under 40 years of age. The distribution of vessel involvement in children parallels that of adults, with diffuse aortic involvement predominating. Signs and symptoms include hypertension, cardiomegaly, elevated ESR, fever, fatigue, palpitations, vomiting, nodules, abdominal pain, arthralgia, claudication, weight loss, and chest pain.

PHYSICAL EXAMINATION

This is particularly helpful in light of the need to completely suppress the vasculitis in order to prevent disease progression. Laboratory markers may be entirely normal despite ongoing inflammation, so MRI offers a potentially more sensitive test for residual disease.

LABORATORY

During the early phases of the disease, markers of systemic inflammation correspond with active vasculitis. Later in the process, vascular lesions may progress in the absence of elevated ESR, CRP, or platelets, significantly complicating treatment aimed at fully controlling disease activity.

IMAGING

Angiography has been the standard method used for diagnosing TA. The size of the vessels involved and the spotty nature of the vascular inflammation make biopsies impractical. CT and MR angiograms have supplanted traditional angiograms as the modalities of choice (**181–185**). They are less invasive, and MRI offers the opportunity to monitor disease activity by revealing evidence of ongoing vessel wall inflammation. PET scanning may similarly allow simultaneous visualization of disease anatomy and physiology.

DIFFERENTIAL DIAGNOSIS

Different conditions must be considered depending on the presenting complaints of a patient with TA. Fever and systemic inflammation or other non-specific presentations of TA have an enormous differential diagnosis. Loss of peripheral pulses, on the other hand, generates a more restricted list, especially in children. A thorough and thoughtful history and physical examination is the most important element in making the accurate diagnosis.

PROGNOSIS

As with all vasculitides, early diagnosis and aggressive therapy are important in TA in order to prevent irreversible vessel damage with resulting compromise of vital organs. The delay in diagnosis in children is notably longer than that reported in most adult patient series (19 months in a recent report), possibly explaining the 33% mortality rate, significantly higher than that in adult series.

MANAGEMENT

Steroids as well as the typical immunosuppressive agents used in other vasculitides (including cyclophosphamide, methotrexate, and azathioprine) have shown variable efficacy in TA. A recent report in adults with TA from the Cleveland Clinic documented a high response rate to use of TNF inhibitors. Before starting these, however, it is important to test patients for tuberculosis, since aortitis is associated with mycobacterial infections, especially in less developed countries.

COMPLICATIONS

Organ ischemia may occur secondary to vascular damage. Hypertension may develop for many reasons. Potential complications related to therapy include avascular necrosis and opportunistic infection with corticosteroids. Immunosuppressive medications are also associated with increased risk of opportunistic infections.

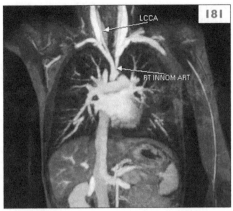

181 Great vessel MRI in Takayasu arteritis.

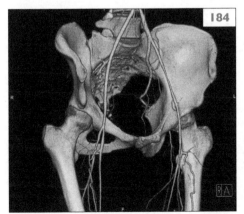

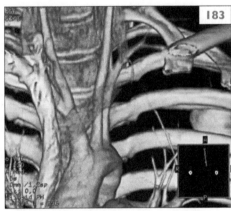

182 Loss of blood flow in the femoral arteries and development of collateral blood flow in Takayasu arteritis.

183 Left brachial artery narrowing in Takayasu arteritis (courtesy of Ann M. Reed MD, Mayo Clinic).

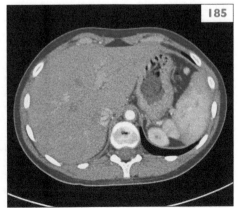

184, 185 Internal femoral artery narrowing in Takayasu arteritis (courtesy of Ann M. Reed, MD, Mayo Clinic) (**184**); Takayasu arteritis – thickened aorta (courtesy of Ann M. Reed, MD, Mayo Clinic) (**185**).

Primary angiitis of the central nervous system

DEFINITION
Primary angiitis of the central nervous system (PACNS) is an inflammatory vasculopathy that is limited to cerebral vessels. It was originally described in adults in 1959, and diagnostic criteria were proposed in 1992. These same criteria, stressing the development of neurologic deficits in someone without a systemic condition that can account for the findings, are used in children as well.

EPIDEMIOLOGY AND ETIOLOGY
The frequency with which isolated CNS vasculitis occurs in children is unknown because of its novelty; it may go unrecognized by practitioners who are not aware that such an entity exists. In adults, PACNS is estimated to have an incidence of 2–3 cases per 1,000,000 person-years. In the largest pediatric series, boys represented 61% of cases.

Rare cases of CNS vasculitis following varicella have been recognized for decades, and in many cases a preceding infection appears to trigger the condition. In most cases, however, children are diagnosed with PACNS without a convincing environmental, infectious, or genetic explanation.

Biopsies of children with PACNS typically demonstrate lymphocytic infiltration of the wall of cerebral vessels (**186**). Adults typically have necrotizing granulomas that are not commonly seen in children. These findings suggest an ongoing immunologic attack against an unidentified antigen, though whether this represents true autoimmunity or a response to an exogenous agent is not known.

CLINICAL HISTORY
Headache (80%) and focal neurologic deficits (78%) are the most common presenting complaints in children diagnosed with PACNS of the large- or medium-sized cerebral vessels, followed by hemiparesis in 62% (**187**). Though small-vessel disease may present with the same findings, such patients are more likely to have systemic complaints such as fever or malaise as well. Global CNS dysfunction is uncommon, though children may have seizures or gradual cognitive decline.

PHYSICAL EXAMINATION
A thorough neurologic exam is essential in any child suspected of having CNS vasculitis. Small- vessel disease is commonly multifocal, so patients often have subtle evidence of isolated abnormalities of strength or sensation of which they may not even be aware. A patient examiner may also detect cranial neuropathies, optic neuritis, or myelitis.

LABORATORY
In PACNS, acute-phase reactants are typically normal, and examination of CSF might be unrevealing as well. Even when a patient has abnormal laboratory studies, they tend to be non-specific, such as elevated serum acute-phase reactants, CSF pleocytosis, or increased intracranial pressure. Thus, diagnosis depends on demonstration of vascular abnormalities on imaging or biopsy.

IMAGING
Brain and cerebral vessel imaging are indicated in any child with CNS abnormalities that cannot be ascribed to a clearly defined infectious, toxic, or vascular abnormality. A normal MR scan together with normal CSF have a high negative predictive value for PACNS. None-the-less in 5–10% of cases, only a meningeal and brain biopsy, guided by clinical or MRI abnormalities or performed blindly, is diagnostic of CNS vasculitis.

DIFFERENTIAL DIAGNOSIS
The differential diagnosis includes the following:
• Infectious process
• Atherosclerosis
• Embolic disease
• Systemic vasculitits
• Toxin/drug
• Malignancy
• Systemic autoimmune disorder.

PROGNOSIS
The number of pediatric cases of isolated CNS vasculitis is insufficient to generate useful prognostic information. Further, an unknown but significant minority of children with PACNS, especially those with localized medium- or large-vessel disease, appear to recover without therapy. It is clear, however,

that early recognition and treatment are essential to ensure optimal outcomes.

MANAGEMENT

Brain biopsy is indicated in many children with suspected PACNS, both to confirm the diagnosis and to exclude mimics of CNS vasculitis, especially atypical infections that could worsen if immunosuppression is started empirically. PACNS may be rapidly progressive and neurologically devastating, so risks of diagnostic procedures must be weighed against the need for prompt diagnosis and initiation of therapy. Treatment includes corticosteroids as well as a potent immunosuppressive agent, usually cyclophosphamide. Once remission is achieved, patients are often switched to methotrexate or azathioprine for maintenance therapy.

COMPLICATIONS

CNS sequelae depend on the area of brain involved. Potential complications related to therapy include avascular necrosis and opportunistic infection with corticosteroids. Immunosuppressive medications are also associated with increased risk of opportunistic infections.

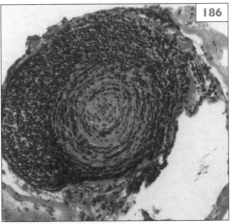

186 Lymphocytic vascular infiltrate in a child with CNS vasculitis (courtesy of Bryce Binstadt, MD, PhD).

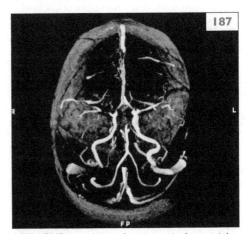

187 CNS vasculitis as hemiparesis due to right parietal infarct from diffuse vascular narrowing (courtesy of Bryce Binstadt, MD, PhD).

Scleroderma in children

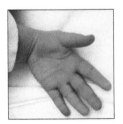
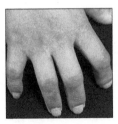
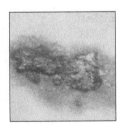
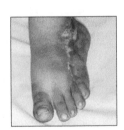

Scleroderma in children includes a group of multisystem autoimmune conditions with the unifying characteristic of the presence of hard skin and the onset before 16 years of age. They may be classified into two main categories: juvenile systemic sclerosis (JSSc) and juvenile localized scleroderma (JLS), known also as morphea.

Juvenile systemic sclerosis

DEFINITION

Juvenile systemic sclerosis (JSSc) is a chronic, multisystem, connective tissue disease characterized by symmetric thickening and hardening of the skin, associated with fibrous changes in internal organs, such as the esophagus, intestinal tract, heart, lungs, and kidneys, arthritis, and myositis. Very recently, a Committee on Classification Criteria for JSSc, including pediatricians, rheumatologists, and dermatologists, developed new classification criteria (Zulian et al. 2007b). On the basis of these criteria, a patient, aged younger than 16 years, shall be classified as having JSSc if the one major criterion, presence of proximal skin sclerosis/induration, and at least 2 of 20 minor criteria, grouped in nine main categories, are present (Table 26).

EPIDEMIOLOGY AND ETIOLOGY

In general, systemic sclerosis (SSc) has an estimated annual incidence ranging from 0.45 per 100,000 to 1.9 per 100,000, and a prevalence of approximately 15–24 per 100,000 (Mayes et al. 2003). Onset in childhood is very uncommon: children under 16 years account for less than 5% of all cases (Scalapino et al. 2006) and fewer than 10% develop SSc before the age of 20 (Black 1999, Kornreich et al. 1977, Medsger 1994). The onset occurs at a mean age of 8.1 years and the peak age is between 10 and 16 years (Martini et al. 2006, Scalapino et al. 2006). The disease is almost four times more frequent in females and there is no racial predilection (Martini et al. 2006).

The cause of SSc is unknown despite significant advances in the understanding of the pathogenic mechanisms since its initial description (Jimenez & Derk 2004). The disease can be represented as a tripartite process in which dysfunction of the immune system, endothelium, and fibroblasts gives rise to a heterogeneous phenotype that is characterized prominently by fibrosis.

Autoimmunity is evident by the elaboration of circulating disease-specific autoantibodies. Fibroblast dysfunction is manifested as fibrosis due to increased synthesis and deposition of extracellular matrix proteins. Raynaud phenomenon, capillary dropout, endothelial injury, and abnormalities in vascular tone are manifestations of endothelial cell dysfunction. These three aspects, although apparently unrelated to each other, are, actually, closely linked by several immunologic alterations.

The excessive accumulation of collagen in affected skin has led to the hypothesis that there may be abnormalities of collagen type or metabolism (Jelaska et al. 1996). Many reports suggest that cellular immunity plays a major role in the initiation of scleroderma. Several cytokines are increased in scleroderma serum including IL-1, IL-2, IL-4, IL-6, and IL-8 (Atamas et al. 1999, Hasegawa et al. 1999) (Table 27). Endothelial cell injury is another important pathogenic event and often predates fibrotic changes in scleroderma.

Table 26
Classification criteria for juvenile systemic sclerosis

Major criterion	Proximal sclerosis/induration of the skin
Minor criteria	
Skin	Sclerodactyly
Vascular	Raynaud phenomenon
	Nailfold capillary abnormalities
	Digital tip ulcers
Gastrointestinal	Dysphagia
	Gastroesophageal reflux
Renal	Renal crisis
	New-onset arterial hypertension
Cardiac	Arrhythmias
	Heart failure
Respiratory	Pulmonary fibrosis (HRCT/radiograph) D$_{LCO}$
	Pulmonary hypertension
Musculoskeletal	Tendon friction rubs
	Arthritis
	Myositis
Neurologic	Neuropathy
	Carpal tunnel syndrome
Serology	ANA
	SSc selective autoantibodies (anti-centromere, anti-topoisomerase I, anti-fibrillarin, anti-PM-Scl, anti-fibrillin, or anti-RNA polymerase I or III)

A patient, aged younger than 16 years, shall be classified as having juvenile systemic sclerosis if the one major criterion and at least 2 of the 20 minor criteria are present. This set of classification criteria has a sensitivity of 90%, a specificity of 96%, and a kappa statistic value of 0.86.

Table 27
Cytokines in juvenile systemic sclerosis

Cytokine/growth factor	Biologic effect
TGF-β, PDGF, IL-1, IL-4, IL-6	Increased collagen synthesis
IFN-β, IFN-γ, TNF-α, β	Decreased collagen synthesis
IFN-β, IFN-γ, TGF-β, PDGF, TNF, IL-1, IL-4	Fibroblasts proliferation
IFN-γ, TGF-β, PDGF, TNF, IL-4	Chemoattraction
TGF-β, TNF, IL-1	Glycosaminoglycan synthesis
TGF-β, IL-4	Fibronectin synthesis
IFN-γ, TNF-α, β, IL-2, NK cell, granzyme A	Endothelial cell injury
TGF-β	Reduction of synthesis
TNF-α	Collagenase gene induction

TGF, transforming growth factor; IFN, interferon; PDGF, platelet-derived growth factor.

CLINICAL HISTORY

The clinical features at the onset of the disease include mainly Raynaud phenomenon and skin induration (**188**). Raynaud phenomenon is the first sign of the disease in 70% of patients and in 10% it is complicated by digital infarcts. Raynaud phenomenon is more common in the fingers (**189**) but can be observed in the toes, ears, lips, tongue, and tip of the nose. Proximal skin induration develops later and is the second most frequent symptom, being present in around 40% of patients at onset (Martini *et al.* 2006).

Other presenting complaints include arthralgia, arthritis, and, although less frequently, muscle weakness, dyspnoea, and calcinosis. Unlike adults, telangiectasia is rarely present in children with JSSc.

PHYSICAL EXAMINATION

Cutaneous involvement in JSSc includes nailfold changes as well as skin induration. These nailfold capillary changes are reported in 40% of patients but their frequency could be much higher if nailfold evaluation was regularly done (Martini *et al.* 2006). Raynaud phenomenon, positive ANA, and the presence of capillaroscopy changes represent the early signs of the disease and precede by months or years the onset of the other clinical features. These unspecific findings identify the so-called 'pre-scleroderma' status (LeRoy & Medsger 2001). Cutaneous changes characteristically evolve in a sequence beginning with edema, followed by induration resulting in marked tightening and contracture (**190–192**). The skin becomes waxy in texture, tight, hard, and bound to subcutaneous structures. This is particularly noticeable in skin of the digits and face where the characteristic expressionless appearance of the skin may be the first clue to diagnosis (**193**). Distal tuft loss can seen on radiographs with severe vasospasm (**194**).

In children with JSSc, visceral organ involvement can be widespread and is associated with significant morbidity. GI involvement may occur in 30–70% of children with JSSc. Most affected patients have esophageal dysfunction, resulting in gastroesophageal reflux (GER) and dysphagia. Manometry, esophageal scintigraphy, and intraesophageal 24-hour pH monitoring provide more sensitive indicators of diminished lower esophageal sphincter tone and GER (Weber *et al.* 2000). Large bowel involvement is less frequent and presents as alternating complaints of constipation and diarrhea, bloating, or abdominal discomfort. Lactulose breath test to evaluate bacterial overgrowth, endoscopy, or colon scintigraphy is a useful tool to evaluate this portion of intestinal tract.

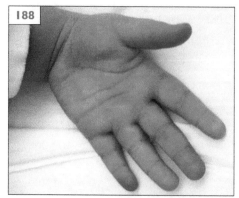

188 Classic Raynaud phenomenon in a 4-year-old girl. Note the ischemic changes (blanching phase) of the second and fourth fingers and the cyanosis (bluish phase) of the fifth finger.

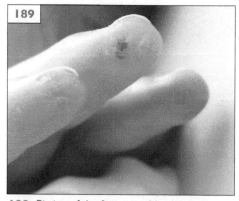

189 Pitting of the fingertips. Note a small ulceration of the tip of the right third finger and shiny, tightly stretched skin over the fingertips.

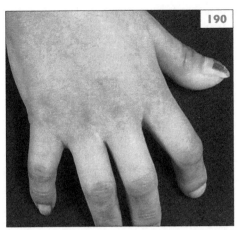

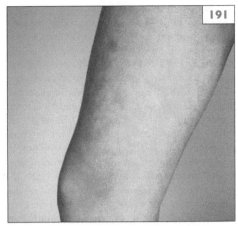

190, 191 Tightness of the skin and early mottling in a new-onset patient. (courtesy of Ann M. Reed, MD, Mayo Clinic).

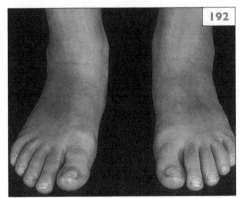

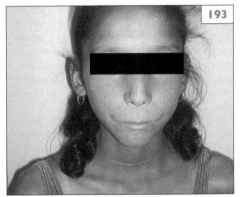

192 Tightness of the skin and early mottling in a new-onset patient. (courtesy of Ann M. Reed, MD, Mayo Clinic).

193 Classic expressionless appearance of a 10-year-old girl with systemic sclerosis. Note also the waxy, translucent appearance of the skin in the upper trunk (courtesy of Dr Ruben Cuttica, Buenos Aires).

194 Distal tuft loss of the first and second DIP joints in a 10-year-old girl with systemic sclerosis and severe sclerodactyly and Raynaud phenomenon (courtesy of Ann M. Reed, MD, Mayo Clinic).

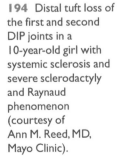

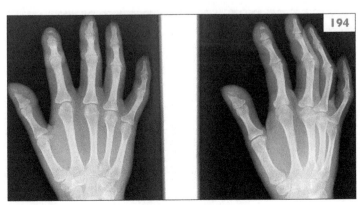

Pulmonary involvement, although frequently asymptomatic, can be present as a dry, hacking cough to dyspnea on exertion. Unlike adults, interstitial pulmonary fibrosis is not frequently reported in children with JSSc at onset but may develop later on during the course of the disease (**195**). Other abnormalities can be pleuritis, abnormal DLCO and pulmonary arterial hypertension (Martini *et al.* 2006, Scalapino *et al.* 2006). The classic radiographic features of interstitial lung disease consist of symmetric, reticulonodular shadowing, most pronounced at the lung bases. High-resolution CT (HRCT) may reveal pulmonary disease even in the presence of a normal chest radiograph. In children, HRCT findings include ground-glass opacification, subpleural micronodules, linear opacities, and honeycombing (Koh & Hansell 2000, Seely *et al.* 1998). In addition, DLCO and spirometry are sensitive measures of involvement of the respiratory tract. Pulmonary vascular disease occurs very rarely, either as a primary event or as a result of pulmonary fibrosis. In this case, echocardiography is an important tool in detecting early pulmonary hypertension, which should be confirmed by right heart catheterization.

Cardiac involvement is present in around one-fifth of the patients and represents a primary cause of morbidity among children with JSSc (Foeldvari *et al.* 2000, Martini *et al.* 2009, Scalapino *et al.* 2006). Pericardial effusions are not common and are usually of no hemodynamic significance. In addition, pulmonary hypertension caused by pulmonary vascular disease can lead to myocardial damage and right heart failure. Cardiorespiratory complications are the leading cause of death in children with JSSc (Foeldvari *et al.* 2000, Martini *et al.* 2009, Scalapino *et al.* 2006).

There are limited data on the prevalence of renal involvement in children with JSSc. In children with SSc, about 10% had some kind of renal involvement including either increased urinary protein excretion or raised creatinine level (Martini *et al.* 2006, Scalapino *et al.* 2006). Although renal involvement in children appears to be not so severe and frequent as in adults, the abrupt onset of accelerated hypertension with acute renal failure (scleroderma renal crisis) remains one of the most severe and life-threatening complications of JSSc.

LABORATORY

About a quarter of JSSc patients have anemia of chronic disease, or, less commonly, macrocytic anemia due to malabsorption. Leukocytosis is not prominent but correlates with the degree of visceral or muscle disease. Patients with myositis have elevated levels of creatine kinase (Martini *et al.* 2006, Scalapino *et al.* 2006). High titers of ANAs are commonly found in 80–90% of children with JSSc (Martini *et al.* 2006, Scalapino *et al.* 2006). The prevalence of both anti-topoisomerase I (Scl-70) and ACA, SSc-specific antibodies, is lower in children compared with adults, being present in 34% and 7% of the patients, respectively (Martini

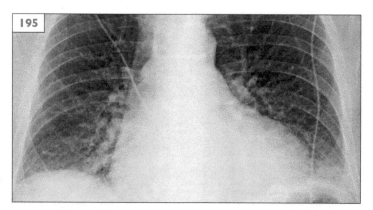

195 Imaging of pulmonary interstitial fibrosis in systemic sclerosis (courtesy of Ann M. Reed, MD, Mayo Clinic).

et al. 2006). Positive RF is present in 17% of patients and correlates with the presence of articular involvement (Martini *et al.* 2006).

IMAGING
Imaging is not a prominent tool for managing the skin involvement of JSSc. Joint radiography may help in the assessment of arthritis. Chest imaging, including CT may be needed to evaluate potential interstitial lung disease. Contrast-based GI studies may be utilized to assess potential esophageal disease.

DIFFERENTIAL DIAGNOSIS
Primary Raynaud phenomenon is not associated with any organ involvement. While few other conditions are associated with skin induration, when this occurs in the hands (as it frequently does), it can be confused with an evolving inflammatory arthropathy. Also, particularly when other organ involvement is noted, other connective tissue diseases, such as SLE, are in the differential diagnosis.

PROGNOSIS
Generally, the prognosis of JSSc is poor. Skin tightness and joint contractures inevitably lead to severe disability (Bottoni *et al.* 2000). It has been reported that the skin may eventually soften years after onset of the disease. Survivorship has not been determined in any large series of children because of the rarity of this disease and very few retrospective data are available (Foeldvari *et al.* 2000, Martini *et al.* 2009, Scalapino *et al.* 2006). The overall mortality rate at 5 years ranges between 6% and 15% and is better than in adults. The causes of death in JSSc include cardiac failure (67%), end-stage renal failure (13%), respiratory failure (10%), infections (7%), and hypertensive encephalopathy (3%) (Foeldvari *et al.* 2000, Martini *et al.* 2009).

MANAGEMENT
Due to the rarity of SSc in children, very little information is available on the treatment and no controlled studies have been performed so far. The non-pharmacologic measures include physiotherapy to help maintain functional ability, muscle strength, and joint movement while preventing flexion contractures, and the use of corrective splints to treat or prevent contractures. Patients and parents should be told to avoid cold and trauma since they can exacerbate symptoms.

The pharmacologic management of patients with JSSc is challenging since no drug has been shown to be of significant benefit in either children or adults with SSc. Calcium channel blockers, usually oral nifedipine or nicardipine, should be considered as first-line therapy for Raynaud phenonemon, and iloprost, or other available IV prostanoids, for severe SSc-related Raynaud phenonemon and digital ulcers (Pope *et al.* 1998, Zulian *et al.* 2004). In accordance with the data for adults, cyclophosphamide may be considered for the treatment of SSc-related interstitial lung disease in children (Hoyles *et al.* 2006, Tashkin *et al.* 2006).

Since steroids seem to be associated with a higher risk of scleroderma renal crisis (DeMarco *et al.* 2002, Steen & Medsger 1998), patients on steroids, for concomitant myositis or arthritis, should be carefully monitored for blood pressure and renal function.

Methotrexate, which is widely used for the treatment of many rheumatic conditions in children, has been shown to improve skin softening in adults (Pope *et al.* 2001) and could be the treatment of choice for skin manifestations also for children, especially in the early phase of the disease.

New drugs for the treatment of pulmonary arterial hypertension, such as bosentan, sitaxsentan, and sildenafil, have been recently introduced in adult patients with SSc (Barst *et al.* 2004, Galie *et al.* 2005, Rubin *et al.* 2002). There is limited experience, at present, to recommend their use in children.

COMPLICATIONS
The most common causes of death in children are related to involvement of the cardiac, renal, and pulmonary systems. Cardiomyopathy, although rare, can be one of the causes of early death, especially in children (Quartier *et al.* 2002). Interstitial lung disease and renal failure or acute hypertensive encephalopathy supervenes as a potentially fatal outcome in few children and seems more likely to occur early in the disease course (Foeldvari *et al.* 2000, Martini *et al.* 2009). Complications of medical therapies such as infections associated with immunosuppressive medications and bone disease related to corticosteroids may occur.

Juvenile localized scleroderma

DEFINITION

Juvenile localized scleroderma (JLS), known as morphea, comprises a group of conditions that involve essentially the skin and subcutaneous tissues. They have various features and range from very small plaques to extensive fibrotic lesions which may cause significant functional and cosmetic deformity.

EPIDEMIOLOGY AND ETIOLOGY

Although JLS is relatively uncommon, it is far more common than SSc in childhood, by a ratio of at least 10:1 (Peterson *et al.* 1997). There is a mild female predilection, the F:M ratio being 2.4:1 (Zulian *et al.* 2006a). The disease onset is usually during late infancy although a few cases with onset at birth have been described (Zulian *et al.* 2006b).

The etiology and pathogenesis of localized scleroderma (LSc) remain uncertain. Two possible contributing pathogenic processes include abnormal fibroblast function and autoimmune dysfunction. One study demonstrated increased collagen production by fibroblasts in skin biopsy specimens from patients with morphea (Kähäri *et al.* 1988). In addition, raised levels of cytokines that increase collagen synthesis by fibroblasts have been reported in LSc lesions (Liu & Connolly 1998). Autoantibodies are a frequent finding in patients with LSc (Harrington & Dunsmore 1989, Liu & Connolly 1998, Zulian *et al.* 2006a). Relatives of affected patients also have an increase in organ-specific autoantibodies compared with control patients (Harrington & Dunsmore 1989). In a large multicenter retrospective review of 750 patients, 13.3% of the patients reported specific environmental events as a potential trigger for their disease (Zulian *et al.* 2006a). These included infections, drugs, mechanical events (e.g. accidental trauma, insect bite, and vaccination), and psychological stress. Trauma has been implicated in the initiation of morphea lesions in 3–13% of patients with LSc (Harrington & Dunsmore 1989, Liu & Connolly 1998, Zulian *et al.* 2006a). The underlying mechanisms on how trauma would contribute to the development of LSc is unclear, although cytokines and neuropeptides (e.g. endothelin-1), which are normally involved in wound healing, have been suggested to play a causative role (Liu & Connolly 1998).

CLINICAL HISTORY

The primary presentation of JLS is dermatologic. Skin lesion(s) may develop in any skin area. They are generally painless, and may be expanding. Other features depend on what area of skin is involved. If the lesion is on the trunk, it may be completely asymptomatic or a change in skin color or texture. If the lesion occurs on the face, it will likely be noticed earlier in the disease course. The family may notice different skin color and texture of the child's face, or facial movements may seem altered. If the lesion occurs on an extremity, it could impact the range of motion (ROM) of the underlying joint. The classification of JLS is based on clinical and pathologic findings discussed below.

PHYSICAL EXAMINATION

JLS can be classified into five subtypes: circumscribed morphea, linear scleroderma, generalized morphea, pansclerotic morphea, and a mixed subtype where a combination of two or more of the previous subtypes is present (*Table 28*). Circumscribed morphea is characterized by oval or round circumscribed areas of induration surrounded by a violaceous halo. It is confined to the dermis with only occasional involvement of the superficial panniculus. Sometimes, as in deep morphea, the entire skin feels thickened, taut, and bound down (**196a, 196b**).

Table 28
Classification criteria of juvenile localized scleroderma (Consensus conference, Padua (Italy) 2004)

Main group	Subtype	Description
Circumscribed morphea	Superficial	Oval or round circumscribed areas of induration limited to epidermis and dermis, often with altered pigmentation and violaceous, erythematous halo (lilac ring). They can be single or multiple
	Deep	Oval or round circumscribed deep induration of the skin involving subcutaneous tissue extending to fascia and may involve underlying muscle. The lesions can be single or multiple. Sometimes the primary site of involvement is in the subcutaneous tissue without involvement of the skin
Linear scleroderma	Trunk/limbs	Linear induration involving dermis, subcutaneous tissue, and, sometimes, muscle and underlying bone and affecting the limbs and/or the trunk
	Head	*En coup de sabre* (ECDS). Linear induration that affects the face and/or the scalp and sometimes involves muscle and underlying bone Parry–Romberg syndrome (or progressive hemifacial atrophy): loss of tissue on one side of the face that may involve dermis, subcutaneous tissue, muscle, and bone. The skin is mobile
Generalized morphea		Induration of the skin starting as individual plaques (four or more and larger than 3 cm) that become confluent and involve at least two anatomic sites
Pansclerotic morphea		Circumferential involvement of limb(s) affecting the skin, subcutaneous tissue, muscle, and bone. The lesion may also involve other areas of the body without internal organ involvement
Mixed morphea		Combination of two or more of the previous subtypes. The order of the concomitant subtypes, specified in brackets, will follow their predominant representation in the individual patient, i.e. mixed (linear-circumscribed)

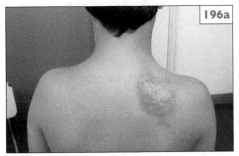 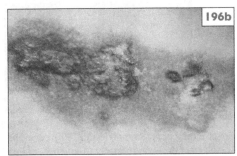

196a Circumscribed morphea in a 12-year-old boy: single indurate plaque with evident hyperemic border ('lilac ring').

196b Circumscribed morphea with keloid formation after biopsy.

When individual plaques are four or more, larger than 3 cm and become confluent, we have the so-called generalized morphea (**197–200**). Linear scleroderma, the most common subtype in children and adolescents, is characterized by one or more linear streaks that can extend through the dermis, subcutaneous tissue, and muscle to the underlying bone, causing significant deformities (**201–206**).

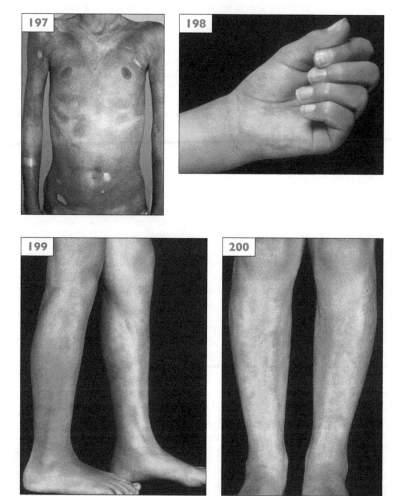

197–200 Generalized morphea in a 17-year-old male: indurate plaques that become confluent and involve the trunk symmetrically (**197**); generalized morphea in a girl with new-onset disease, which resolved entirely on treatment (courtesy of Ann M. Reed, MD, Mayo Clinic) (**198**); generalized morphea in a girl with new-onset disease, which resolved entirely on treatment (courtesy of Ann M. Reed, MD, Mayo Clinic) (**199**); generalized morphea in a girl with new-onset disease, which resolved entirely on treatment (courtesy of Ann M. Reed, MD, Mayo Clinic) (**200**).

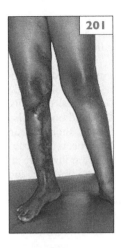

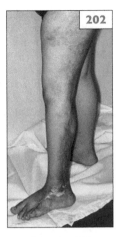

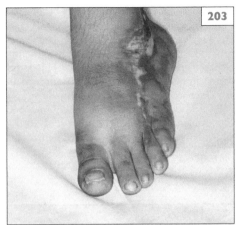

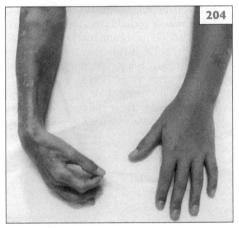

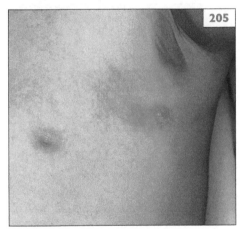

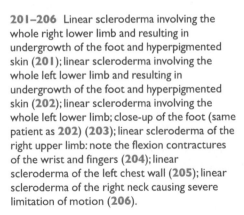

201–206 Linear scleroderma involving the whole right lower limb and resulting in undergrowth of the foot and hyperpigmented skin (**201**); linear scleroderma involving the whole left lower limb and resulting in undergrowth of the foot and hyperpigmented skin (**202**); linear scleroderma involving the whole left lower limb; close-up of the foot (same patient as **202**) (**203**); linear scleroderma of the right upper limb: note the flexion contractures of the wrist and fingers (**204**); linear scleroderma of the left chest wall (**205**); linear scleroderma of the right neck causing severe limitation of motion (**206**).

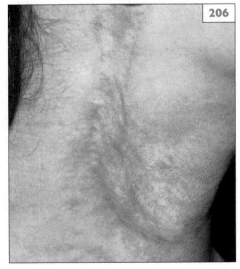

The upper or lower extremities can be affected but also face or scalp, as in the *en coup de sabre* (ECDS) variety so called because the lesion looks like the depression caused by a dueling stroke from a sword (**207–211**). This latter form can be complicated by CNS abnormalities, such as calcifications, vasculitis or simply MRI-unspecific abnormalities, and dental and even ocular abnormalities (Zannin *et al.* 2007). In patients with ECDS, associated neurologic manifestations include seizures (particularly complex partial seizures), headaches, and facial paralysis. The neurologic findings may occur before, concurrent with, or after the skin manifestations. Parry–Romberg syndrome (or progressive hemifacial atrophy) loss of tissue on one side of the face that may involve dermis, subcutaneous tissue, muscle, and bone is also seen (**210, 211**). Pansclerotic morphea, an extremely rare but severe subtype, is characterized by generalized full-thickness involvement of the skin of the trunk, extremities, face, and scalp with sparing of the fingertips and toes (**212**). Eosinophilic fasciitis is a form that extends into the fascia with inflammation and eosinophils present with boggy, tight extremities (**213, 214**).

Extracutaneous manifestations in patients with LSc mainly include articular, neurologic, ocular, and GI involvement (Zulian *et al.* 2005). Articular involvement is the most frequent finding, being reported in 19% of the patients (Dehen *et al.* 1994, Zulian *et al.* 2005). It is mainly present in patients with linear scleroderma. These children tend to have an accelerated course with predominant musculoskeletal disease, including rapid development

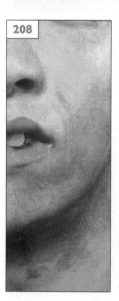

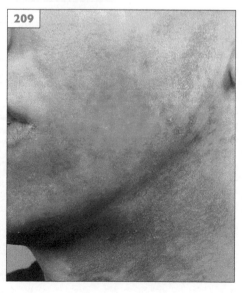

207–209 Linear scleroderma ECDS affecting the left forehead and resulting in two lines of induration, hyperpigmentation, and depression of the scalp in varying stages and individuals (courtesy of Ann M. Reed, MD, Mayo Clinic).

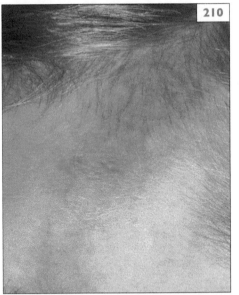
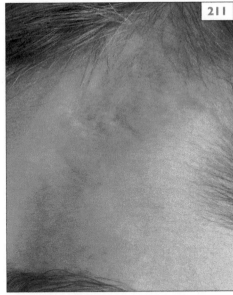
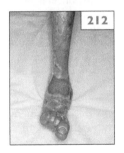
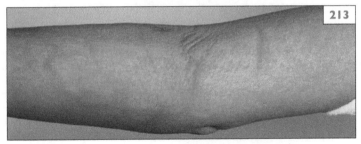

210–214 Linear scleroderma and Parry–Romberg syndrome (or progressive hemifacial atrophy) loss of tissue on one side of the face that may involve dermis, subcutaneous tissue, muscle and bone (courtesy of Ann M. Reed, MD, Mayo Clinic) (**210, 211**); disabling pansclerotic morphea (**212**); eosinophilic fasciitis in a young girl on presentation (courtesy of Ann M. Reed, MD, Mayo Clinic) (**213, 214**).

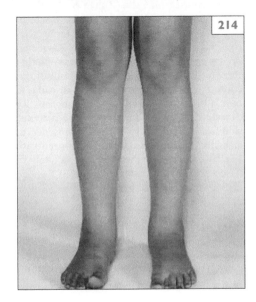

of contractures. Neurologic manifestations, reported in 4% of the patients, consist essentially in epilepsy and headaches, behavioral changes, and learning disabilities (Blaszczyk et al. 2003, Kister et al. 2008, Zulian et al. 2005). Abnormalities on MRI, such as calcifications, white matter changes, vascular malformations, and changes consistent with CNS vasculitis, have also been reported (Kister et al. 2008). Ocular changes are reported in 3.2% of the children affected by localized scleroderma (Zannin et al. 2007). As expected, most of them have ECDS but, interestingly, around one-third had no facial skin lesion. The most frequent lesions are on eyelids and eyelashes, one-third consisting of anterior segment inflammation, such as anterior uveitis or episcleritis, the remaining being CNS-related abnormalities, paralytic strabismus, pseudopapilledema, or refractive errors.

Esophageal motor function abnormalities with GER have been reported in 2–4% of children with JLS (Guariso et al. 2007, Zulian 2004). These findings might support the indication for an extensive GI evaluation in patients with LSc, especially in the presence of specific GI symptoms.

LABORATORY

In a large cohort of patients, ANAs were found in 42% of patients with no correlation between their presence and a particular subtype or disease course (*Table 29*) (Zulian et al. 2006a). Anti-topoisomerase I antibodies (anti-Scl-70) and ACAs, specific markers of systemic sclerosis, were found to be positive in 2–3% of children with JLS (Zulian et al. 2006a). Whether these antibodies reflect just the immunologic component of the disease process or can also have a prognostic significance is unclear. RF detected, at low titre in 16% of the patients, significantly correlates with the presence of arthritis (Zulian et al. 2006a). Children with LSc who develop arthritis are more likely to have a positive RF, and sometimes an elevated ESR and circulating autoantibodies (Zulian et al. 2005).

IMAGING

The management of JLS is challenging and the detection of disease activity and progression remains a fundamental problem. Non-invasive technology may be helpful in following the extent of disease in selected patients. Thermography, which measures the radiation of infrared heat from the body, is able to discriminate active from inactive lesions (Martini et al. 2002). This procedure is non-invasive and usually well tolerated. It allows for easy interpretation and rapid results that are helpful in decision-making. There are false-positive results in cases of atrophic or old lesions, particularly in the scalp region (Martini et al. 2002).

Ultrasonography is a non-invasive tool, which may also be useful in the evaluation of LSc patients (Cosnes et al. 2003). Unfortunately, this evaluation is difficult in overweight patients, operator dependent, and not yet standardized for children. Ultrasonography can also be used to monitor disease activity (Li et al. 2007). A computerized skin score method allows the measurement of single target lesions and comparison over time. It consists in the demarcation of the indurate borders of the lesions on an adhesive transparent film and subsequent transfer, as a scanned image, in a computer (Zulian et al. 2007a). The calculation of the affected area is then performed by computer software. This new technique is applicable in day-to-day practice, is not time-consuming, and does not need specialized equipment.

Bone growth malformations may be monitored with radiographs to determine bone maturation and possible surgical intervention (**215**).

Table 29 Serum autoantibodies in juvenile localized scleroderma		
Serum autoantibody	Patients %	Healthy controls %
ANA	42.3	0–3
Anti-topoisomerase I	3.2	0
ACA	1.7	0
Anti-dsDNA	4.2	0
RF	16	0–4
APL antibody	12.6	1.5–9.4

DIFFERENTIAL DIAGNOSIS

Other dermatologic conditions, such as vitiligo, are in the differential diagnosis of JLS. When it occurs over a peripheral joint(s), it can be confused with an inflammatory arthropathy. When presentation includes facial involvement, particularly in a young child, consideration of congential abnormalities is given.

PROGNOSIS

The prognosis of JLS depends primarily on what area of the skin is involved. Facial disease, and skin inolvment over peripheral joints may have greater consequences if disease progresses. Also, if the JLS involves deeper skin layers, it is frequently more difficult to treat.

MANAGEMENT

Over the years, many treatments have been tried for localized scleroderma. Unfortunately, the rarity of the disease and the difficulty in assessing outcomes in an objective way have limited the interpretation of most of these studies.

Treatment should be mainly topical such as moisturizing agents, topical glucocorticoids, or calcipotriene (Cunningham *et al.* 1998). When there is a significant risk for disability, such as in linear and deep subtypes, systemic treatment with methotrexate in combination with corticosteroids should be considered (Uziel *et al.* 2000, Weibel *et al.* 2006). Methotrexate can be used at a weekly regimen of 10–15 mg/m^2 as a single oral or subcutaneous dose for at least 1 year. During the first 2–3 months of therapy, a course of glucocorticoid steroids (prednisone 0.5–1 mg/kg per day administered orally or methylprednisolone 20–30 mg/kg per day administered intravenously for three consecutive days) may be used as adjunctive bridge therapy for those with rapidly progressive disease. Most patients show a response within 2–4 months and the side effects are usually mild and associated more with corticosteroid than with methotrexate treatment. Unfortunately, no controlled trials are available and the series of treated patients are very small.

COMPLICATIONS

Circumscribed morphea generally is of cosmetic concern only, and frequently lesions spontaneously remit with residual pigmentation as the only abnormality. With ECDS, facial disfigurement can occur. Rarely seizure disorders can be associated with this form of JLS. Persistient flexion contractures of peripheral joints may be seen as well. Complications of medical therapies such as infections associated with immunosuppressive medications and bone disease related to corticosteroids may occur.

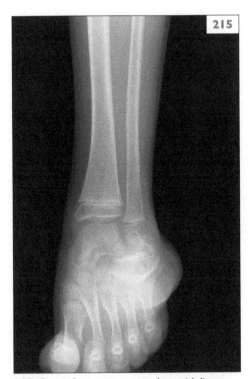

215

215 Bone changes in a young boy with linear scleroderma (courtesy of Ann M. Reed, MD, Mayo Clinic).

Autoinflammatory diseases

- The monogenic autoinflammatory diseases
- Other monogenic autoinflammatory syndromes

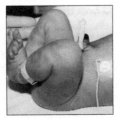
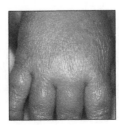
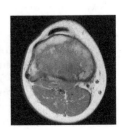

The autoinflammatory diseases or the periodic fever syndromes have opened a new chapter in the field of rheumatology. The systemic autoinflammatory diseases are a group of rare disorders characterized by unprovoked inflammatory episodes without high-titer autoantibodies (Stojanov & Kastner 2005). These are mainly monogenic diseases where mutations in a single gene in the inflammatory pathway have been associated with a disease. The most typical example is familial Mediterranean fever (FMF). However, recently a number of other complex diseases have been included in this group (Ozen et al. 2006).

THE MONOGENIC AUTOINFLAMMATORY DISEASES

Familial Mediterranean fever

DEFINITION
Familial Mediterranean fever (FMF, MIM249100) is a disease caused by mutations in the gene coding for pyrin (Aksentijevich et al. 1999). Clinically it is characterized by recurrent attacks of fever and serositis along with increased acute-phase inflammation (Samuels & Ozen 2006).

EPIDEMIOLOGY AND ETIOLOGY
The disease is caused by mutations in the Mediterranean fever (*MEFV*) gene. Mutations in this gene are known to be very common in people of eastern Mediterranean origin with carrier rates as high as 1:3 to 1:5 (Yilmaz et al. 2001). The frequency of these mutations has led to investigations on the advantage introduced by the carrier state for these mutations. Today it is widely believed that these mutations offer a better and maybe exaggerated inflammatory response to pathogens (Lachmann et al. 2006, Ozen et al. 2002).

More than 50 mutations in the *MEFV* gene have been associated with FMF (Aksentijevich et al. 1999, Stojanov & Kastner 2005). The *MEFV* gene consists of 10 exons and most of the disease-causing mutations are located on exon 10.

The gene codes for pyrin, an important protein of the inflammasome and the inflammatory pathway. Pyrin regulates IL-1 produc-tion through its interaction with caspase-1; a direct effect of pyrin on IL-1β activation and the idea that pyrin interacts directly with caspase-1 to modulate IL-1β production has been suggested in recent studies (Chae et al. 2006). Thus mutations in pyrin are associated with increased IL-1β production. In fact the IL-1 receptor antagonist anakinra was shown to suppress acute-phase proteins in a patient with FMF and amyloidosis (Chae et al. 2006).

CLINICAL HISTORY
The hallmark of clinical presentation is the typical attacks in the form of fever and serositis along with elevation in acute-phase reactants (Samuels & Ozen 2006). The typical attack of FMF lasts half a day to 3 days, and is accompanied by fever (Livneh et al. 1996). Myalgia may occur (Tunca et al. 2005). In the majority of patients serositis manifests itself as abdominal pain. The pain is incapacitating. Arthritis and/or arthralgia is also very frequent and is present in half of the patients in the large series reported from Israel and Turkey (Livneh et al. 1996, Tunca et al. 2005). Pleurisy in the form of chest pain is common; it is unilateral and often spreads to the shoulder.

The disease is clinically diagnosed on the basis of typical attacks with increased inflammatory response. Livneh et al., from Israel, have suggested a set of criteria for diagnosis; however, these have not been validated in other ethnic groups (Livneh et al. 1997). According to these criteria there are major and minor criteria as well as supportive criteria. The four major criteria include the typical attacks (≥ 3 of the same type; rectal temperature $\geq 38°C$; 12–72 hour) with peritonitis, pleuritis, monoarthritis (hip, knee, and ankle), and fever alone. Minor criteria are defined as incomplete attacks, exertional leg pain, and favorable response to colchicines (Livneh et al. 1997).

PHYSICAL EXAMINATION
The only skin manifestation of FMF – except when it is associated with vasculitis – is erysipelas-like erythema (ELE), which is provoked by pressure-bearing exercise (**216**). ELE may not necessarily accompany an attack. In fact some manifestations of FMF are not associated with an attack. These include protracted febrile myalgia, hematuria, arthralgia, and exertional myalgia. Another

interesting feature of FMF is the association with vasculitides and especially polyarteritis nodosa (Ozen *et al.* 2001). A large series from Turkey has shown that these patients have increased rates of Henoch–Schönlein purpura, polyarteritis nodosa, and probably Behçet disease (Tunca *et al.* 2005).

LABORATORY

Subclinical inflammation persists even in between attacks (Lachmann *et al.* 2006). Lachmann *et al.* have shown that there was also some inflammatory activity between attacks as well (median SAA 6 mg/l, CRP 4 mg/l). They have thus suggested that substantial subclinical inflammation occurs widely and over prolonged periods in patients with FMF, indicating that the relatively infrequent clinically overt attacks represent the 'tip of the iceberg' in this disorder.

IMAGING

Imaging is not compulsory in diagnosing FMF. An ultrasound and chest radiograph may show fluid in the peritoneum and pleura, respectively. An echocardiogram may demonstrate pericardial fluid in rare cases who have pericarditis.

DIFFERENTIAL DIAGNOSIS

A mutation analysis for the *MEFV* gene is indicated in a patient who has recurrent attacks lasting less than 3 days with elevated acute-phase reactants, and lacks any skin findings except for ELE and lacks the features of the other periodic fever diseases (*Table 30*). The ethnic background is important in the differential workup of these patients, though one must not forget that FMF patients have been identified in many ethnic groups including Japanese individuals. Differential diagnosis includes all other periodic fever syndromes and is very problematic in a patient who does not have an eastern Mediterranean ancestry (*Table 30*) (Samuels & Ozen 2006). Urticaria and other skin findings that occur in other periodic fever syndromes are not present in FMF. The time frame of the attack helps in differentiating from TRAPS. However, the most important differentiating characteristic of FMF is probably the response to colchicine. This is the rationale for using colchicine for a trial period in patients who are thought to have FMF but lack genetic confirmation.

PROGNOSIS

This is the only periodic fever where an excellent quality of life is possible in the majority of patients – with a cheap pill. In fact colchicine has been shown to prevent amyloidosis in compliant patients in series from Israel and Turkey (Kallinich *et al.* 2007, Saatci *et al.* 1997, Zemer *et al.* 1991). Colchicine is also indicated for quality of life since it prevents attacks or decreases the severity and/or frequency of attacks (Kallinich *et al.* 2007).

MANAGEMENT

Evidence for the effectiveness of colchicine in children suffering from FMF came from subsequently performed open-label studies (evidence level IIA) (Kallinich *et al.* 2007). In the large cohorts of children (*n* = 809) no manifestation of amyloidosis occurred in 809 treated children during an observation period of up to 13 years (Zemer *et al.* 1991). In the Turkish FMF registry 2.3% developed amyloidosis, all being non-compliant with respect to regular colchicine intake (Saatci *et al.* 1997).

A starting dose of colchicine 0.5 mg/day in young children and 1.0 mg/day in older children (>5 years) is sufficient for disease control in approximately half of patients (evidence level IIB) (Kallinich *et al.* 2007). The dose is increased to the adult dose of 1.5–2 mg/day once the child weighs more than 27 kg. High SAA levels might indicate insufficient disease control and thereby the need for

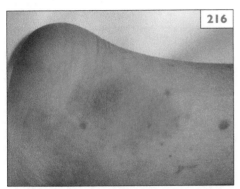

216 Erysipelas-like erythema in a child with FMF.

dose adjustment (evidence level III) (Kallinich et al. 2007).

There are many problems that as pediatricians we should warn the families about: the risk in any other children; to follow the siblings closely for any symptoms of unexplained fever or typical attacks. A routine mutation analysis of the *MEFV* gene for sibs is probably not indicated. However, if there is a case of renal amyloidosis in the family, a genetic workup may be required. SAA levels may also be checked in siblings.

The diagnosis in a patient without genetic confirmation is more problematic. Since this is an autosomal recessively inherited disease we require the presence of two mutations in the *MEFV* gene to confirm the diagnosis of FMF. However, there may be patients who resemble the FMF phenotype but have failed to show two or even any mutation in the *MEFV* gene. A trial of colchicine is warranted if the patient has a phenotype suggestive of FMF since this is the only autoinflammatory disease that responds to colchicine. A trial with and without colchicine should be compared in terms of attacks and acute-phase response, especially the SAA levels. Features of other autoinflammatory diseases should be carefully sought out, especially in patients who do not have an eastern Mediterranean ancestry.

COMPLICATIONS

The primary potential complication of FMF is the development of amyloidosis. Complications of colchicine treatment include diarrhea.

Table 30
Differential diagnosis of periodic fevers

	FMF	HIDS
Inheritance[a]	Recessive	Recessive
Predominant ethnicities/ ancestries	Jewish, Armenian, Arab, Turkish, Italian	Dutch, French, other Europe
Gene	*MEFV*	*MVK*
Protein	Pyrin (marenostrin)	Mevalonate kinase
Duration of episodes	1–3 days	3–7 days
Cutaneous disease	Erysipeloid-like erythema	Skin rash or eruptions, rare HSP
Musculoskeletal findings	Episodic monoarthritis, sacroiliitis	Arthralgia, non-erosive polyarthritis
Abdominal involvement	Sterile peritonitis 85%	Pain, emesis, diarrhea; peritonitis uncommon
Other key features	Pleurisy, asymptomatic pericardial effusions; scrotal pain	Cervical adenopathy, elevated IgD, elevated urinary mevalonate during attack
Treatment	Colchicine prophylaxis	NSAIDs, for arthritis (anecdotal anti-TNF-α, statins)

[a]Inheritance patterns are all autosomal.

(with permission from Samuels & Ozen 2006)

TRAPS	FCAS	MWS	NOMID/CINCA	PAPA
Dominant	Dominant	Dominant	Dominant	Dominant
Irish and Scottish, but expanding	Mostly European	Northern European	None	None
TNFRSF1A	*CIAS1/NALP3/ PYPAF1*	*CIAS1/NALP3/ PYPAF1*	*CIAS1/NALP3/ PYPAF1*	*PSTPIP1/ CD2BP1*
55 dDa TNF receptor	Cryopyrin	Cryopyrin	Cryopyrin	PSTPIP1/CD2BP1
Often >1 week	Usually <24 hours	24–48 hours	Continuous but with flares	Variable
Migratory erysipelas-like rash overlying myalgias	Urticarial rash induced by exposure to cold	Urticarial rash	Urticarial rash	Pyoderma gangrenosum, acne
Severe migratory myalgia, arthralgia, often non-erosive monoarthritis	Myalgias, debilitating polyarthralgias	Myalgias, intermittent arthralgias, large joint oligoarticular arthritis	Epiphyseal/patellar overgrowth, periosteal elevation, intermittent or chronic arthritis	Pyogenic, sterile arthritis
Pain, peritonitis, diarrhea, constipation	Nausea	Pain	Uncommon but hepatosplenomegaly with flares	None
Pleurisy	Headache	Sensorineural deafness	Learning disability, chronic aseptic meningitis, headache, senorineural deafness	Destructive, recurrent inflammation in skin, joints, and muscles
Anti-TNF-α prophylaxis	Avoidance of cold, anti-IL-1, NSAIDs	Anti-IL-1, NSAIDs, prednisone?	Anti-IL-1, anecdotal anti-TNF-α	Steroids (anecdotal anti-IL-1 and anti-TNF)

Cold-induced autoinflammatory syndrome 1 (CIAS1-pathies) – the cryopyrin-associated periodic fever syndromes

DEFINITION

The cryopyrin-associated periodic fever syndromes (CAPS) include familial cold autoinflammatory syndrome (FCAS, MIM120100), Muckle–Wells syndrome (MWS, MIM191900), and neonatal-onset multisystem inflammatory disease (NOMID, also known as chronic infantile neurologic cutaneous articular (CINCA) syndrome, MIM607115).

Cold-induced autoinflammatory syndrome 1 (CIAS1), CIAS1-pathies or cryopyrinopathies, or CAPS, is a group of autoinflammatory diseases caused by mutations in the gene coding for cryopyrin (Samuels & Ozen 2006, Stojanov & Kastner 2005). In this group we have three major diseases, with FCAS representing the mildest and NOMID the most severe form of the disease complex (Hawkins *et al.* 2004, Hoffman *et al.* 2004, Johnstone *et al.* 2003, Neven *et al.* 2004).

EPIDEMIOLOGY AND ETIOLOGY

The reported patients with FCAS and MWS have been mainly confined to European ancestry whereas NOMID/CINCA has been reported in a variety of ethnic groups (Stojanov & Kastner 2005). A negative family history in NOMID suggests new mutations in this serious disease.

Cryopyrin shares a similar pyrin domain. Cryopyrin forms a macromolecular complex with ASC, CARDINAL (CARD8), and caspase-1 called the inflammasome, which mediates caspase-1 and IL-1β activation (Ozen *et al.* 2006, Stojanov & Kastner 2005). Mutations in cryopyrin are believed to cause an increased inflammasome activity.

Although these three syndromes may be associated with different mutations in CIAS1 and there is some phenotype–genotype correlation, the same single missense mutation can produce variant phenotypes and/or overlapping phenotype with partial criteria from two or more of these syndromes (Hawkins *et al.* 2004, Hoffman *et al.* 2004, Johnstone *et al.* 2003, Neven *et al.* 2004). There is considerable overlap among some patients and there is evidence that other genes and/or environmental factors are effective in the pathogenesis of these diseases.

CLINICAL HISTORY

All of the CIAS1-pathies are characterized by fevers and a non-pruritic, urticarial rash (**217–221**) usually presenting in infancy (later in MWS), and they may have some overlapping features as described below. FCAS presents with attacks precipitated by cold as suggested in the name. The main differentiating feature of MWS is the hearing defect. The naming of the third disease in this group reflects the characteristics of the disease: NOMID for the onset and CINCA for the involved systems. NOMID and sometimes the other diseases tend to have more persistent features and may lack the typical attacks that may prove important in the differential diagnosis (Samuels & Ozen 2006).

PHYSICAL EXAMINATION

There are some overlapping signs such as conjunctivitis (FCAS, MWS) or sensorineural hearing loss and systemic amyloidosis (MWS, NOMID) among these diseases. Unique features of each disease include the precipitation of attacks by generalized cold exposure in FCAS, the hearing defect in MWS and more severe CNS involvement including optic nerve irritation/papilledema, chronic aseptic meningitis, learning disability, as well as facial dysmorphia in NOMID (Hawkins *et al.* 2004, Hoffman *et al.* 2004, Johnstone *et al.* 2003, Neven *et al.* 2004). The musculoskeletal involvement can be in the form of arthralgias (FCAS) to synovitis (MWS) to the characteristic arthropathy of NOMID/CINCA with premature ossification and overgrowth and bone inflammation (**222**). The arthropathy of NOMID/CINCA is very characteristic.

LABORATORY

There are no specific laboratory tests. Acute-phase reactants are expected to be increased.

IMAGING

Imaging may be useful to identify bony abnormalities including inflammation and overgrowth (**223**) and to exclude other causes of periodic fevers.

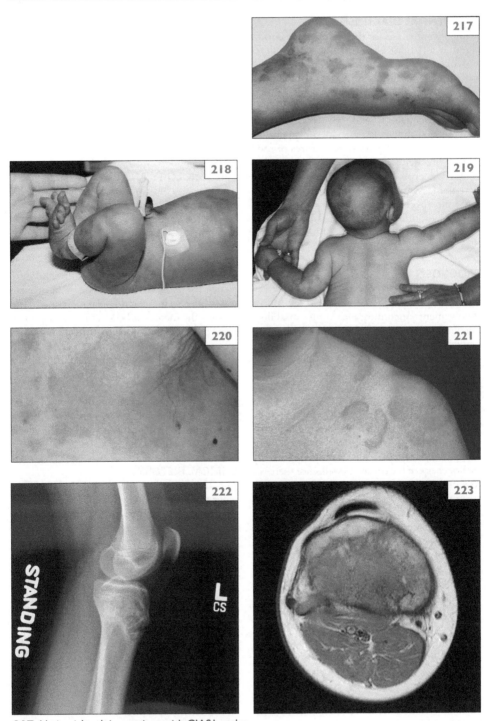

217 Urticarial rash in a patient with CIAS1-pathy.
218–223 Urticarial rash in a newborn with CIAS1-pathy (courtesy of Ann M. Reed, MD, Mayo Clinic) (**218, 219**); urticarial rash as seen in a patient with FCAS and MWS (courtesy of Dawn Davis, MD, Mayo Clinic) (**220, 221**); bone lesions seen in CIAS1-pathy (courtesy of Ann M. Reed, MD, Mayo Clinic) (**222, 223**).

DIFFERENTIAL DIAGNOSIS

A mutation analysis for the CIAS1 gene is indicated in a patient with inflammatory attacks provoked by cold – even air conditioning, a patient with hearing loss and recurring attacks with urticaria unresponsive to colchicine, or a young feverish child with recurrent meningitis or other neurologic and skin features. The differential diagnosis includes all other periodic fever syndromes. The unique features of each disease are helpful. It should be noted that NOMID is probably the only disease with more persistent symptoms rather than attacks. Systemic juvenile idiopathic arthritis and a number of infectious diseases may also be considered in the differential diagnosis of NOMID/CINCA.

PROGNOSIS

NOMID/CINCA represents the most severe condition and can be complicated with CNS involvement including learning disability, chronic aseptic meningitis, increased intracranial pressure, papilledema, cerebral atrophy, and sensorineural hearing loss as well as chronic inflammatory and destructive arthropathy, skeletal dysplasia, and retinal dystrophy.

MANAGEMENT

Case reports and open-label studies highlight the success of anti-IL-1 treatment currently with anakinra (Lovell *et al.* 2005). This fits in with the pathogenesis of the disease as well since there is a loss of control in IL-1 production. Anti-IL-1 treatment has even been effective in suppressing amyloidosis. Symptomatic treatment and avoidance of cold are also important for FCAS. There are case reports with etanercept (only versus the arthropathy) as well (Federico *et al.* 2003).

COMPLICATIONS

Secondary amyloidosis may occur as a complication of ongoing inflammation. Opportunistic infections may occur with anti-IL-1 therapy.

Hyperimmunoglobulinemia D with periodic fever syndrome

DEFINITION

Hyperimmunoglobulinemia D with periodic fever syndrome (HIDS, MIM260920) is an autosomal recessively inherited periodic fever syndrome caused by mutations in the gene *MVK*, which codes for the enzyme mevalonate kinase (Drenth *et al.* 1999).

EPIDEMIOLOGY AND ETIOLOGY

The majority of the reported patients are from the Netherlands and France. However, cases have been reported worldwide. The lack of mevalonate causes an elevation of mevalonic acid along with a lack of production of the downstream elements, which are the isoprenoids (Frenkel *et al.* 2001). The deficiency of isoprenoids has been shown to contribute to increased IL-1β secretion. Thus it is not the increased IgD but rather the metabolic pathway that leads to the inflammatory burst (Frenkel *et al.* 2001, Ozen *et al.* 2006). HIDS is actually a milder form of the disease named mevalonic aciduria, which results in even higher levels of urinary mevalonate. Those children have mutations on the same gene as HIDS but suffer from severe neurologic deficits and dysmorphic features as well as the fevers (Prietsch *et al.* 2003).

CLINICAL HISTORY

The attacks typically last for 2–7 days. They recur without obvious periodicity. Along with the fever, abdominal pain, diarrhea, and vomiting are common (Frenkel *et al.* 2001, Prietsch *et al.* 2003). Arthralgia is common. The attacks may be provoked by vaccinations as well. The severity of symptoms varies among patients and tends to be milder as the child grows (Drenth *et al.* 1999, Frenkel *et al.* 2001).

PHYSICAL EXAMINATION

Along with the fever hepatosplenomegaly and cervical lymphadenopathy are seen (Frenkel *et al.* 2001, Prietsch *et al.* 2003). Arthritis may be noted. Rashes are present in three-quarters of the patients (**224**).

LABORATORY
There is leukocytosis and increased acute-phase reactants during attacks. Serum IgD levels are usually elevated during attacks; however, this is not a prerequisite for the diagnosis and it may be elevated in other autoinflammatory diseases as well (Frenkel *et al.* 2001). On the other hand, as a result of the mevalonate kinase deficiency there is an increased excretion of urinary mevalonic acid and this may be a helpful differentiating feature.

IMAGING
Imaging may be useful to exclude other causes of periodic fevers.

DIFFERENTIAL DIAGNOSIS
A mutation analysis of the *MVK* gene is indicated in a patient (especially from Dutch or French ancestry) with recurring attacks of fever and pain not responding to colchicine, who also has cervical lymphadenopathy, and some rash that lasts less than a week. Diagnosis depends on characteristic features with high serum IgD and high urine mevalonate levels. For genetic confirmation mutations need to be shown on the *MVK* gene. All inherited periodic fevers and especially PFAPA syndrome should be considered in the differential diagnosis (Samuels & Ozen 2006). There is no response to colchicine in HIDS.

PROGNOSIS
The frequency of attacks decreases by age. Although the risk of amyloidosis seems to be low the patients suffer from a poor quality of life in the early years.

MANAGEMENT
We lack a high level of evidence for the treatment of HIDS. Anti-TNF and anti-IL-1 treatment has been reported to be effective in recent papers (Bodar *et al.* 2005). Statins have been tried; however, they did not have a significant effect and had to be stopped in some patients due to side effects (Simon *et al.* 2004b).

COMPLICATIONS
There has been only one case of amyloidosis.

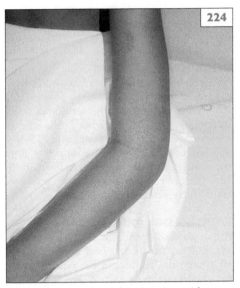

224 Maculopapular rash in a patient with HIDS.

Tumor necrosis factor receptor-associated periodic syndrome

DEFINITION

Mutations on chromosome 12 in TNFRSF1A, the gene encoding the 55-kDa receptor for TNF has been associated with the autosomal dominantly inherited disease, tumor necrosis factor receptor-associated periodic syndrome (TRAPS, MIM142680) (McDermott *et al.* 1999). Both the number of known mutations (more than 30) and the spectrum of affected ethnicities have considerably increased over the last years.

EPIDEMIOLOGY AND ETIOLOGY

Although first defined in Scottish and Irish individuals, patients have now been diagnosed all around the world and the syndrome can occur in any ethnic group (Ozen *et al.* 2006, Stojanov & Kastner 2005).

In healthy controls, TNF-α activates TNFRSF1A receptors and releases these receptors from the cell surface to be shed into the extracellular compartment. The unattached TNF receptors are free to bind TNF-α and reduce the cellular inflammatory response to it (McDermott *et al.* 1999). In most of the patients with TRAPS there is a shedding defect in the aforementioned receptor (Stojanov & McDermott 2005). However, recent findings suggest that the shedding hypothesis does not account for all cases.

Thus a more complex mechanism may be involved in at least some of the patients (Ozen *et al.* 2006, Stojanov & Kastner 2005).

The pedigree is compatible with an autosomal dominant inheritance.

CLINICAL HISTORY

Patients have prolonged (greater than 1 week) attacks of fever associated with abdominal pain, and myalgia.

PHYSICAL EXAMINATION

Patients may have an erythematous skin rash (**225a**), conjunctivitis, and/or periorbital edema (Hull *et al.* 2002, McDermott 1999). Muscle involvement is a frequent feature in these patients, usually involving only one muscle group at a time. Myalgia has been shown to frequently result from monocytic fasciitis, but also from myositis or lymphocytic vasculitis.

LABORATORY

Acute-phase reactants are elevated as in other periodic fever syndromes.

IMAGING

Imaging may be useful to exclude other causes of periodic fevers.

DIFFERENTIAL DIAGNOSIS

A family history is almost always present. Mutation analysis for the TRAPS gene is indicated in a patient who presents with attacks longer than a week with myalgia or myositis and migratory rashes and with affected cases in the pedigree.

PROGNOSIS
AA amyloidosis develops in 25–40% of patients with TRAPS, with the kidneys and liver being the most common complication.

MANAGEMENT
Understanding the etiology has brought up the logical use of TNF-α inhibition. Case reports and open-label studies confirmed anti-TNF treatment as a safer and more effective alternative to corticosteroid therapy with regard to the frequency, duration, and severity of attacks (Drewe *et al.* 2004). Etanercept may also reverse or slow the clinical progression of renal amyloidosis in TRAPS. However, this may not always be the case. For the rare cases when anti-TNF-α therapy does not work anti-IL-1 therapy may prove useful (Simon *et al.* 2004a).

COMPLICATIONS
Amyloidosis has been reported in these patients; 14% of those reported so far have developed amyloidosis (**225b**). Thus urinalysis needs to be checked at each visit. Amyloidosis has been associated with cysteine substitutions (Hull *et al.* 2002).

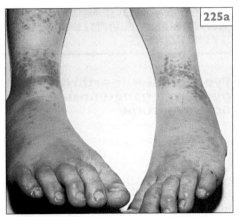

225a Fasciitis in a patient with TRAPS (courtesy of Dr M. Gattorno).

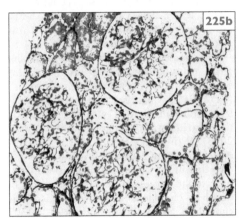

225b Amyloidosis in a renal biopsy of a child with TRAPS.

OTHER MONOGENIC AUTOINFLAMMATORY SYNDROMES

Pyogenic sterile arthritis, pyoderma gangrenosum, and acne syndrome

Pyogenic sterile arthritis, pyoderma gangrenosum, and acne (PAPA) syndrome is a very rare disease, characterized by early destruction of the joints (**226–228**) by recurrent effusions. The patients also experience infiltration of muscle and numerous dermatologic manifestations including cystic acne, expanding purulent ulcerating lesions (pyoderma gangrenosum), and sterile abscesses at injection sites (Lindor *et al.* 1997). It is mainly a white American disease (Stojanov & Kastner 2005). It is inherited in an autosomal dominant fashion.

The disease is caused by mutations in proline serine threonine phosphatase-interacting protein (PSTPIP1, or CD2-binding protein 1 (CD2BP1)), which is a tyrosine-phosphorylated protein involved in cytoskeletal organization, also interacting with pyrin (Shoham *et al.* 2003). Pyrin binds the PSTPIP1/CD2BP1 protein, defining FMF and PAPA syndrome as disorders in the same pathway. Shoham *et al.* have found increased IL-1β production by peripheral blood leukocytes from a patient with clinically active PAPA with the A230T PSTPIP1/CD2BP1 mutation, consistent with the hypothesis that these mutations exert a dominant-negative effect on the previously reported activity of pyrin (Shoham *et al.* 2003, Stojanov & Kastner 2005). The disease is mediated predominantly by granulocytes as in FMF.

While some patients benefit from corticosteroids many of them become resistant to therapy. Biologics (anti-TNF and anti-IL-1) have been tried with varying success in resistant patients (Samuels & Ozen 2006, Stojanov & Kastner 2005).

Early onset sarcoidosis (sporadic granulomatous arthritis), Blau syndrome (familial granulomatous arthritis), and Crohn disease

CARD15 is a caspase recruitment domain; CARD15 serves as an intracellular sensor of bacteria and is another member of the inflammatory pathway leading to the activation of IL-1β. It participates in an inflammatory signaling cascade triggering NF-κB (Rose & Martin 2005). CARD15 mutations have been shown in 40% of patients with Crohn disease, 50% of those with Blau syndrome, and 90% of patients early onset sarcoidosis (EOS). Thus mutations in this protein have been associated with the aforementioned granulomatous (auto-)inflammatory diseases (Stojanov & Kastner 2005).

Blau syndrome is an autosomal, dominantly inherited syndrome characterized by synovitis, uveitis, and rash (**229–231**). The histology of the synovium, conjunctiva, and dermis show the typical non-caseating granuloma (**232**). EOS has similar characteristics but lacks family history. It is now widely accepted that Blau syndrome and EOS are the same disease, with an inherited mutation in Blau syndrome and a new mutation EOS (Rose & Martin 2005). In fact, CARD15 mutations are present in 50% and 90% of Blau syndrome and EOS patients, respectively (Rose & Martin 2005).

CROHN DISEASE

Some patients with Crohn disease also share a mutated form of CARD15. It should be stressed that similar to Blau syndrome, non-caseating granulomas and arthritis may also be found in Crohn disease (Rose & Martin 2005). Arthritis is a feature of this IBD. Understanding more about the pathophysiology may enable us to have more specific therapeutic options in these diseases.

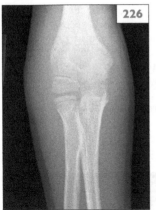

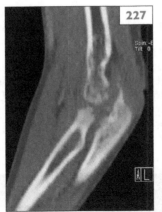

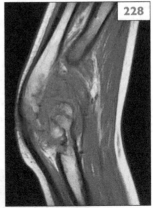

226–228 Destructive arthropathy in PAPA syndrome (courtesy of Ann M. Reed, MD, Mayo Clinic).

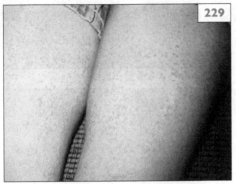

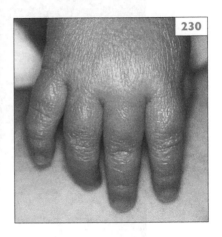

229 Cutaneous skin granulomas in Blau syndrome in adolescence (courtesy of Ann M. Reed, MD, Mayo Clinic).

230–232 Cutaneous skin granulomas in Blau syndrome at birth (courtesy of Ann M. Reed, MD, Mayo Clinic) (**230, 231**); bone granuloma in Blau syndrome (courtesy of Ann M. Reed, MD, Mayo Clinic) (**232**).

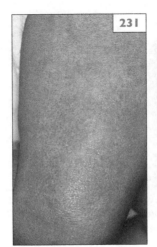

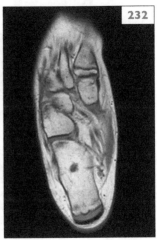

NON-BACTERIAL OSTEITIS

Chronic recurrent multifocal osteomyelitis (CRMO) and synovitis, acne, pustulosis, hyperostosis, and osteitis (SAPHO) syndrome are characterized by recurring attacks of bone pain and fever. The osteomyelitis may recur months or years later (**233–236**). There is an autosomal recessive syndromic form of the disease, called Majeed syndrome, in which the mutated gene is identified (Ferguson *et al.* 2006). A similar, autosomal, recessively inherited mouse model has been identified where there is bone, cartilage, and skin inflammation. In these mice the mutated gene is *PSTPIP2*, which shares significant sequence homology to the *PSTPIP1* (the mutated gene of PAPA syndrome) (Ferguson *et al.* 2006).

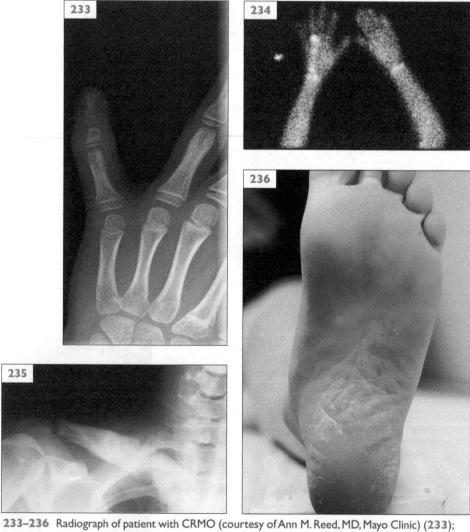

233–236 Radiograph of patient with CRMO (courtesy of Ann M. Reed, MD, Mayo Clinic) (**233**); bone scan of patient with CRMO (courtesy of Ann M. Reed, MD, Mayo Clinic) (**234**); clavicular osteomyelitis in a patient with SAPHO (courtesy of Ann M. Reed, MD, Mayo Clinic) (**235**); skin findings in SAPHO (**236**).

DEFICIENCY OF THE INTERLEUKIN-1-RECEPTOR ANTAGONIST

Deficiency of the IL-1-receptor antagonist (DIRA) presents in the neonatal period and is characterized by pustulosis, periostitis, and sterile osteomyelitis (**237–240**). The illness arises from mutations in the *IL1RN* gene, which results in a non-functional IL-1-receptor antagonist, causing cellular hypersensitivity to the proinflammatory cytokine interleukin-1 (Aksentijevich *et al.* 2009, Reddy *et al.* 2009).

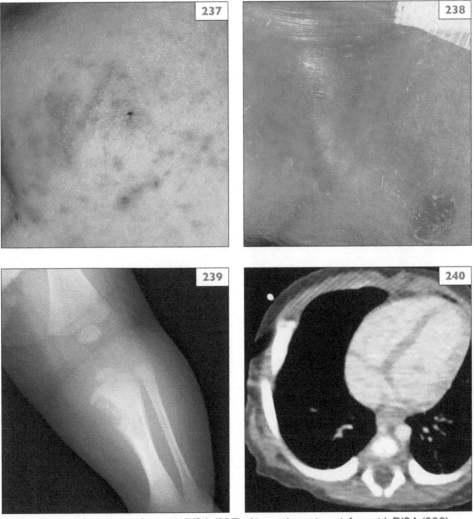

237–240 Pustulosis in an infant with DIRA (**237**); skin erythema in an infant with DIRA (**238**); osteitis in an infant with DIRA (**239**); osteitis of the sixth rib in an infant with DIRA (**240**).

Autoinflammatory syndromes that are not monogenic/ autoinflammatory diseases with complex genetic traits

The spectrum of autoinflammatory syndromes has now been enlarged to include a number of complex genetic syndromes. For example, Behçet syndrome has been suggested to be an autoinflammatory disease since it is characterized by remissions and exacerbations and by an acute-phase response without autoantibodies (Ozen *et al.* 2006). Again, at least a portion of systemic juvenile idiopathic arthritis patients with the high IL-1 levels may be representative of this group. In both of these diseases secondary amyloidosis develops similar to the group of aforementioned monogenic diseases. The group of diseases to be included in this section may expand in future. These diseases do have an autoinflammatory element; however, they have their differentiating features and they require immunosuppressive treatment unlike the typical monogenic diseases.

In conclusion, the autoinflammatory diseases have enlightened our understanding of the pathway of inflammation and innate immunity. Further developments are expected to provide insight into other rheumatic diseases and enable us to manage and treat these patients in a more proper fashion.

References

2. JUVENILE IDIOPATHIC ARTHRITIS

Adib N, Silman A, Thomson W (2005). Outcome following onset of juvenile idiopathic inflammatory arthritis: I. frequency of different outcomes. *Rheumatology (Oxford)*, **44**: 995–1001.

Anthony KK, Schanberg LE (2007). Pediatric pain syndromes and management of pain in children and adolescents with rheumatic disease. *Rheum Dis Clin North Am*, **33**: 625–60.

Arguedas O, Fasth A, Andersson-Gäre B, Porras O (1998). Juvenile chronic arthritis in urban San José, Costa Rica: a 2 year prospective study. *J Rheumatol*, **25**: 1844–50.

Behrens EM, Beukelman T, Paessler M, Cron RQ (2007). Occult macrophage activation syndrome in patients with systemic juvenile idiopathic arthritis. *J Rheumatol*, **34**: 1133–8.

Brewer EJ, Bass JC, Cassidy JT (1972). Criteria for the classification of juvenile rheumatoid arthritis. *Bull Rheum Dis*, **23**: 712–19.

Carrasco R, Smith JA, Lovell D (2004). Biologic agents for the treatment of juvenile rheumatoid arthritis: current status. *Paediatr Drugs*, **6**: 137–46.

Carvounis PE, Herman DC, Cha S, Burke JP (2006). Incidence and outcomes of uveitis in juvenile rheumatoid arthritis, a synthesis of the literature. *Graefes Arch Clin Exp Ophthalmol*, **244**: 281–90.

Cassidy JT, Petty RE, Laxer RM, Lindsley CB (2005). *Textbook of Pediatric Rheumatology*, 5th edn. Elsevier Saunders, Philadelphia, pp. 207, 209.

Cohen SB, Emery P, Greenwald MW, *et al.*; REFLEX Trial Group (2006). Rituximab for rheumatoid arthritis refractory to anti-tumor necrosis factor therapy: results of a multicenter, randomized, double-blind, placebo-controlled, phase III trial evaluating primary efficacy and safety at twenty-four weeks. *Arthritis Rheum*, **54**: 2793–806.

Danner S, Sordet C, Terzic J, *et al.* (2006). Epidemiology of juvenile idiopathic arthritis in Alsace, France. *J Rheumatol*, **33**: 1377–81.

European League Against Rheumatism (1977). *EULAR Bulletin No 4: Nomenclature and Classification of Arthritis in Children*. National Zeitung AG, Basel.

Gäre BA, Fasth A (1992). Epidemiology of juvenile chronic arthritis in southwestern Sweden: a 5-year prospective population study. *Pediatrics*, **90**: 950–8.

Gilliam BE, Chauhan AK, Low JM, Moore TL (2008). Measurement of biomarkers in juvenile idiopathic arthritis patients and their significant association with disease severity: a comparative study. *Clin Exp Rheumatol*, **26**: 492–7.

Habib HM, Mosaad YM, Youssef HM (2008). Anti-cyclic citrullinated peptide antibodies in patients with juvenile idiopathic arthritis. *Immunol Invest*, **37**: 849–57.

Lovell DJ, Giannini EH, Reiff A, *et al.* (2000). Etanercept in children with polyarticular juvenile rheumatoid arthritis. Pediatric Rheumatology Collaborative Study Group. *N Engl J Med*, **342**: 763–9.

Lovell DJ, Ruperto N, Goodman S, *et al.* (2008). Adalimumab with or without methotrexate in juvenile rheumatoid arthritis. *N Engl J Med*, **359**: 810–20.

Malleson PN, Fung MY, Rosenburg AM (1996). The incidence of pediatric rheumatic diseases: results from the Canadian Pediatric Rheumatology Association Disease Registry. *J Rheumatol*, **23**: 1981–7.

Manners PJ, Bower C (2002). Worldwide prevalence of juvenile arthritis why does it vary so much? *J Rheumatol*, **29**: 1520–30.

Martínez Mengual L, Fernández Menéndez JM, Solís Sánchez G, *et al*. (2007). [Epidemiological study of juvenile idiopathic arthritis in the last sixteen years in Asturias (Spain)]. *An Pediatr (Barc)*, **66**: 24–30 [Article in Spanish].

Moe N, Rygg M (1998). Epidemiology of juvenile chronic arthritis in northern Norway: a ten-year retrospective study. *Clin Exp Rheumatol*, **16**: 99–101.

Murray KJ, Moroldo MB, Donnelly P, *et al*. (1999). Age specific effects of juvenile rheumatoid arthritis-associated HLA alleles. *Arthritis Rheum*, **42**: 1843–53.

Oen K, Cheang M (1996). Epidemiology of chronic arthritis in childhood. *Semin Arthritis Rheum*, **26**: 575–91.

Oen K, Malleson PN, Cabral DA, *et al*. (2003). Early predictors of longterm outcome in patients with juvenile rheumatoid arthritis: subset-specific correlations. *J Rheumatol*, **30**: 585–93.

Pascual V, Allantaz F, Patel P, *et al*. (2008). How the study of children with rheumatic diseases identified interferon-alpha and interleukin-1 as novel therapeutic targets. *Immunol Rev*, **223**: 39–59.

Petty RE, Southwood TR, Baum J, *et al*. (1997). Revision of the proposed classification criteria for juvenile idiopathic arthritis: Durban. *J Rheumatol*, **25**: 1991–94, 1998.

Pruunsild C, Uibo K, Liivamägi H, *et al*. (2007). Incidence of juvenile idiopathic arthritis in children in Estonia: a prospective population-based study. *Scand J Rheumatol*, **36**: 7–13.

Quartier P, Taupin P, Bourdeaut F (2003). Efficacy of etanercept for the treatment of juvenile idiopathic arthritis according to the onset type. *Arthritis Rheum*, **48**: 1093–101.

Ruperto N, Lovell DJ, Cuttica R, *et al*. (2007). A randomized, placebo-controlled trial of infliximab plus methotrexate for the treatment of polyarticular-course juvenile rheumatoid arthritis. *Arthritis Rheum*, **56**: 3096–106.

Ruperto N, Lovell DJ, Quartier P, *et al*. (2008). Abatacept in children with juvenile idiopathic arthritis: a randomised, double-blind, placebo-controlled withdrawal trial. *Lancet*, **372**: 383–91.

Sacks JJ, Helmick CG, Luo Y, Ilowite NT (2007). Prevalence of and annual ambulatory health care visits for pediatric arthritis and other rheumatologic conditions in the United States in 2001–2004. *Arthritis Rheum*, **57**: 1439–45.

Schneider R, Laxer RM (1998). Systemic onset juvenile rheumatoid arthritis. *Baillieres Clin Rheumatol*, **12**: 245–71.

Selvaag AM, Lien G, Sørskaar D, *et al*. (2005). Early disease course and predictors of disability in juvenile rheumatoid arthritis and juvenile spondyloarthropathy: a 3 year prospective study. *J Rheumatol*, **32**: 1122–30.

Silverman E, Mouy R, Spiegel L, *et al*. (2005). Leflunomide or methotrexate for juvenile rheumatoid arthritis. *N Engl J Med*, **352**: 1655–66.

Spiegel LR, Schneider R, Lang BA, *et al*. (2000). Early predictors of poor functional outcome in systemic-onset juvenile rheumatoid arthritis: a multicenter cohort study. *Arthritis Rheum*, **43**: 2402–9.

Stoeber E (1981). Prognosis in juvenile chronic arthritis. Follow-up of 433 chronic rheumatic children. *Eur J Pediatr*, **135**: 225–8.

Tristano AG (2008). Macrophage activation syndrome: a frequent but under-diagnosed complication associated with rheumatic diseases. *Med Sci Monit*, **14**: RA27–36.

van Rossum MA, Fiselier TJ, Franssen MJ, *et al*. (1998). Sulfasalazine in the treatment of juvenile chronic arthritis: a randomized, double-blind, placebo-controlled, multicenter study. Dutch Juvenile Chronic Arthritis Study Group. *Arthritis Rheum*, **41**: 808–16.

Wallace CA, Levinson JE (1991). Juvenile rheumatoid arthritis: outcome and treatment for the 1990s. *Rheum Dis Clin North Am*, **17**: 891–905.

Woo P (2006). Systemic juvenile idiopathic arthritis: diagnosis, management, and outcome. *Nat Clin Pract Rheumatol*, **2**: 28–34.

Woo P, Wedderburn LR (1998). Juvenile chronic arthritis. *Lancet*, **351**: 969–73.

Woo P, Wilkinson N, Prieur AM *et al*. (2005). Open label phase II trial of single, ascending doses of MRA in Caucasian children with severe systemic juvenile idiopathic arthritis: proof of principle of the efficacy of IL-6 receptor blockade in this type of arthritis and demonstration of prolonged clinical improvement. *Arthritis Res Ther*, **7**: R1281–8.

3. SPONDYLOARTHROPATHIES AND REACTIVE ARTHROPATHIES

Aggarwal A, Hissaria P, Misra R (2005). Juvenile ankylosing spondylitis – is it the same disease as adult ankylosing spondylitis? *Rheumatol Int*, **25**: 94–6.

Ayoub EM, Ahmed S (1997). Update on complications of group A streptococcal infections. *Curr Probl Pediatr*, **27**: 90–101.

Ayoub EM, Alsaeid K (2005). Acute rheumatic fever and post-streptococcal reactive arthritis. In: Cassidy JT, Petty RE, Laxer RM, Lindsley CB (eds). *Textbook of Pediatric Rheumatology*, 5th edn. Elsevier Saunders, Philadelphia, pp. 614–29.

Baek HJ, Shin KC, Lee YJ, *et al*. (2002). Juvenile onset ankylosing spondylitis (JAS) has less severe spinal disease course than adult onset ankylosing spondylitis (AAS): clinical comparison between JAS and AAS in Korea. *J Rheumatol*, **29**: 1780–85.

Barash J, Mashiach E, Navon-Elkan P, *et al*. (2008). Differentiation of post-streptococcal reactive arthritis from acute rheumatic fever. *J Pediatr*, **153**: 696–9.

Bennett AN, McGonagle D, O'Connor P, *et al*. (2008). Severity of baseline magnetic resonance imaging-evident sacroiliitis and HLA-B27 status in early inflammatory back pain predict radiographically evident ankylosing spondylitis at eight years. *Arthritis Rheum*, **58**: 3413–18.

Burgos-Vargas R (2002). Juvenile onset spondyloarthropathies: therapeutic aspects. *Ann Rheum Dis*, **61**(suppl III): iii33–9.

Burgos-Vargas R, Pacheco-Tena C, Vazquez-Mellado J (1997). Juvenile onset spondyloarthropathies. *Rheum Dis Clin North Am*, **23**: 596–8.

Burgos-Varga R, Vazquez-Mellado J (2005). Reactive arthritis. In: Cassidy JT, Petty RE, Laxer RM, Lindsley CB (eds). *Textbook of Pediatric Rheumatology*, 5th edn. Elsevier Saunders, Philadelphia, pp. 604–13.

Burgos-Vargas R, Vazquez-Mellado J, Cassis N *et al*. (1996). Genuine ankylosing spondylitis in children: a case–control study of patients with early definitive disease according to adult onset criteria. *J Rheumatol*, **23**: 2140–7.

Dajani AS, Ayoub EM, Bierman FZ, *et al.* (1992). Special report: guidelines for the diagnosis of rheumatic fever: Jones criteria, updated 1992: Special Writing Group of the Committee on Rheumatic Fever, Endocarditis, and Kawasaki Disease of the Council on Cardiovascular Disease in the Young of the American Heart Association. *JAMA*, **268**: 2069–73.

Dajani A, Taubert K, Ferrieri P, *et al.* (1995). Treatment of acute streptococcal pharyngitis and prevention of rheumatic fever: a statement for health care professionals. Committee on Rheumatic Fever and Kawasaki disease of the Council on Cardiovascular Disease in the Young, the American Heart Association. *Pediatrics*, **96**(4 Pt 1): 758–64.

Dougados M, van der Linden S, Juhlin R, *et al.* (1991). The European Spondyloarthropathy Study Group preliminary criteria for the classification of spondyloarthropathy. *Arthritis Rheum*, **34**: 1218–27.

Gensler L, Davis J (2006). Recognition and treatment of juvenile-onset spondyloarthritis. *Curr Opin Rheumatol*, **18**: 507–11.

Gensler LS, Ward MM, Reveille JD, *et al.* (2007). Clinical, radiographic and functional differences between juvenile-onset and adult-onset ankylosing spondylitis: results from the PSOAS cohort. *Ann Rheum Dis*, **67**: 233–7.

Hafner R, Michels H (1996). Psoriatic arthritis in children. *Curr Opin Rheumatol*, **8**: 467–72.

Jones TD (1944). The diagnosis of rheumatic fever. *JAMA*, **126**: 481–4.

Kvien TK, Gaston JS, Bardin T, *et al.* (2004). Three month treatment of reactive arthritis with azithromycin: a EULAR double blind, placebo controlled study. *Ann Rheum Dis*, **63**: 1113–19.

Lewkowicz D, Gottlieb AB (2004). Pediatric psoriasis and psoriatic arthritis. *Dermatol Ther*, **17**: 364–75.

Lindsley CB, Laxer RM (2005). Arthropathies of inflammatory bowel disease. In: Cassidy JT, Petty RE, Laxer RM, Lindsley CB (eds). *Textbook of Pediatric Rheumatology*, 5th edn. Elsevier Saunders, Philadelphia, pp. 334–9.

Paiva ES, Macaluso DC, Edwards A, Rosenbaum JT (2000). Characterization of uveitis in patients with psoriatic arthritis. *Ann Rheum Dis*, **59**: 67–70.

Petty RE, Southwood TR (2005). Psoriatic arthritis. In: Cassidy JT, Petty RE, Laxer RM, Lindsley CB (eds). *Textbook of Pediatric Rheumatology*, 5th edn. Elsevier Saunders, Philadelphia, pp. 324–33.

Petty RE, Southwood TR, Manners P, *et al.* (2004). International League of Associations for Rheumatology classification of juvenile idiopathic arthritis: second revision, Edmonton, 2001. *J Rheumatol*, **31**: 390–2.

Prieur AM, Listrat V, Dougados M (1990). Evaluation of the ESSG and the AMOR criteria for juvenile spondyloarthropathies (JSA). Study of 310 consecutive children referred to one pediatric rheumatology center. *Arthritis Rheum*, **33**(suppl 9): S160.

Rosenberg AM (2000). Juvenile onset spondyloarthropathies. *Curr Opin Rheumatol*, **12**: 425–9.

Selvaag AM, Lien G, Sorskaar D, *et al.* (2005). Early disease course and predictors of disability in juvenile rheumatoid arthritis and juvenile spondyloarthropathy: a 3 year prospective study. *J Rheumatol*, **32**: 1122–30.

Stoll ML, Nigrovic PA (2006). Subpopulations within juvenile psoriatic arthritis: a review of the literature. *Clin Dev Immunol*, **13**: 377–80.

Stone M, Warren RW, Bruckel J, *et al.* (2005). Juvenile-onset ankylosing spondylitis is associated with worse functional outcomes than adult-onset ankylosing spondylitis. *Arthritis Rheum*, **53**: 445–51.

van der Linden S, Valkenburg HA, Cats A (1984). Evaluation of diagnostic criteria for ankylosing spondylitis. A proposal for modification of the New York criteria. *Arthritis Rheum*, **27**: 361–8.

van der Linden SM, van der Heijde D, Maksymowych WP (2008). Ankylosing spondylitis. In: Firestein GS, Budd RC, Harris ED, McInnes IB, Ruddy S, Sergant JS (eds). *Kelley's Textbook of Rheumatology*, 8th edn. W. B. Saunders, Philadelphia, pp. 1169–84.

4. LUPUS ERYTHEMATOSUS

Askanase AD, Friedman DM, Copel J, *et al.* (2002). Spectrum and progression of conduction abnormalities in infants born to mothers with anti-SSA/Ro-SSB/La antibodies. *Lupus*, **11**: 145–51.

Barron KS, Silverman ED, Gonzales J, Reveille JD (1993). Clinical, serologic, and immunogenetic studies in childhood-onset systemic lupus erythematosus. *Arthritis Rheum*, **36**: 348–54.

Black C, Isenberg DA (1992). Mixed connective tissue disease – goodbye to all that. *Br J Rheumatol*, **31**: 695–700.

Bohan A, Peter JB (1975a). Polymyositis and dermatomyositis (first of two parts). *N Engl J Med*, **292**: 344–7.

Bohan A, Peter JB (1975b). Polymyositis and dermatomyositis (second of two parts). *N Engl J Med*, **292**: 403–7.

Boros CA, Spence D, Blaser S, Silverman ED (2007). Hydrocephalus and macrocephaly: new manifestations of neonatal lupus erythematosus. *Arthritis Rheum*, **57**: 261–6.

Brucato A, Doria A, Frassi M, *et al.* (2002). Pregnancy outcome in 100 women with autoimmune diseases and anti-Ro/SSA antibodies: a prospective controlled study. *Lupus*, **11**: 716–21.

Brunner H, Silverman E, To T, *et al.* (2002). Risk factors for damage in childhood-onset SLE. *Arthritis Rheum*, **46**: 436–44.

Buyon JP, Hiebert R, Copel J, *et al.* (1998). Autoimmune-associated congenital heart block: demographics, mortality, morbidity and recurrence rates obtained from a national neonatal lupus registry. *J Am Coll Cardiol*, **31**: 1658–66.

Buyon JP, Waltuck J, Caldwell K, *et al.* (1994). Relationship between maternal and neonatal levels of antibodies to 48 kDa SSB(La), 52 kDa SSA(Ro), and 60 kDa SSA(Ro) in pregnancies complicated by congenital heart block. *J Rheumatol*, **21**: 1943–50.

Callen JP (2006). Cutaneous lupus erythematosus: a personal approach to management. *Australas J Dermatol*, **47**: 13–27.

Carreno L, Lopez-Longo FJ, Monteagudo I, *et al.* (1999). Immunological and clinical differences between juvenile and adult onset of systemic lupus erythematosus. *Lupus*, **8**: 287–92.

Cassidy JT, Petty RE (2005). *Textbook of Pediatric Rheumatology*, 5th edn, Elsevier Saunders, Philadelphia, p. xv.

Cimaz R, Spence DL, Hornberger L, Silverman ED (2003). Incidence and spectrum of neonatal lupus erythematosus: a prospective study of infants born to mothers with anti-Ro autoantibodies. *J Pediatr*, **142**: 678–83.

Deapen D, Escalante A, Weinrib L, *et al.* (1992). A revised estimate of twin concordance in systemic lupus erythematosus. *Arthritis Rheum*, **35**: 311–18.

Emre S, Bilge I, Sirin A, *et al.* (2001). Lupus nephritis in children: prognostic significance of clinicopathological findings. *Nephron*, **87**: 118–26.

Fessel WJ (1988). Epidemiology of systemic lupus erythematosus. *Rheum Dis Clin North Am*, **14**: 15–23.

Frankovich J, Sandborg C, Barnes P, *et al.* (2008). Neonatal lupus and related autoimmune disorders of infants. *NeoReviews*, **9**: e206–17.

Gilliam JN, Sontheimer RD (1981). Distinctive cutaneous subsets in the spectrum of lupus erythematosus. *J Am Acad Dermatol*, **4**: 471–5.

Hallengran CS, Nived O, Surfelt G (2004). Outcome of incomplete systemic lupus erythematous after 10 years. *Lupus*, **13**: 85–8.

Hochberg MC (1997). Updating the American College of Rheumatology revised criteria for the classification of systemic lupus erythematosus [letter]. *Arthritis Rheum*, **40**: 1725.

Kasukawa R (1987). Preliminary diagnostic criteria for classification of mixed connective tissue diease. In: Kasukawa R, Sharp GC (eds). *Mixed Connective Tissue Disease and Antinuclear Antibodies*. Elsevier, Amsterdam, pp. 41–47.

Lee LA, Sokol RJ, Buyon JP (2002). Hepatobiliary disease in neonatal lupus: prevalence and clinical characteristics in cases enrolled in a national registry. *Pediatrics*, **109**: E11.

Manzi S, Meilahn EN, Rairie JE, *et al*. (1997). Age-specific incidence rates of myocardial infarction and angina in women with systemic lupus erythematosus: comparison with the Framingham Study. *Am J Epidemiol*, **145**: 408–15.

Martin V, Lee LA, Askanase AD, *et al*. (2002). Long-term followup of children with neonatal lupus and their unaffected siblings. *Arthritis Rheum*, **46**: 2377–83.

Michels H (1997). Course of mixed connective tissue disease in children. *Ann Med*, **29**: 359–64.

Mier RJ, Shishov M, Higgins GC, *et al*. (2005). Pediatric-onset mixed connective tissue disease. *Rheum Dis Clin North Am*, **31**: 483–96.

Mukerji B, Hardin JG (1993). Undifferentiated, overlapping, and mixed connective tissue diseases. *Am J Med Sci*, **305**: 114–19.

Patel P, Werth V (2002). Cutaneous lupus erythematosus: a review. *Dermatol Clin*, **20**: 373–85.

Prendiville JS, Cabral DA, Poskitt KJ, *et al*. (2003). Central nervous system involvement in neonatal lupus erythematosus. *Pediatr Dermatol*, **20**: 60–7.

Ravelli A, Ruperto N, Martini A (2005). Outcome in juvenile onset systemic lupus erythematosus. *Curr Opin Rheumatol*, **17**: 568–73.

Rus VH, Hochberg MC (2002). The epidemiology of systemic lupus erythematous. In: Wallace DJ, Hahn BH (eds). *Dubois' Lupus Erythematosus*, 6th edn, Williams & Wilkins, Baltimore.

Shanske AL, Bernstein L, Herzog R (2007). Chondrodysplasia punctata and maternal autoimmune disease: a new case and review of the literature. *Pediatrics*, **120**: e436–41.

Smolen JS, Steiner G (1998). Mixed connective tissue disease: to be or not to be? *Arthritis Rheum*, **14**: 768–77.

Szyper-Kravitz M, Marai I, Shoenfeld Y (2005). Coexistence of thyroid autoimmunity with other autoimmune diseases: friend or foe? Additional aspects on the mosaic of autoimmunity. *Autoimmunity*, **38**: 247–55.

Tan EM, Cohen AS, Fries JF, *et al*. (1982). The 1982 revised criteria for the classification of systemic lupus erythematosus. *Arthritis Rheum*, **25**: 1271–7.

Tebbe B, Orfanos CE (1997). Epidemiology and socioeconomic impact of skin disease in lupus erythematosus. *Lupus*, **6**: 96–104.

Tiddens HA, van der Net JJ, de Graeff-Meeder ER, *et al*. (1993). Juvenile-onset mixed connective tissue disease: longitudinal follow-up. *J Pediatr*, **122**: 191–7.

Tucker LB, Menon S, Schaller JG, Isenberg DA (1995). Adult- and childhood-onset systemic lupus erythematosus: a comparison of onset, clinical features, serology, and outcome. *Br J Rheumatol*, **34**: 866–72.

Weening JJ, D'Agati VD, Schwartz MM, *et al*. (2004). The classification of glomerulonephritis in systemic lupus erythematosus revisited. *J Am Soc Nephrol*, **15**: 241–50.

Woo P, Laxer RM, Sherry DD (eds) (2007). Systemic lupus erythematosus. In: *Pediatric Rheumatology in Clinical Practice*. Springer, London.

Worrall JG, Snaith ML, Batchelor JR, Isenberg DA (1990). SLE: a rheumatological view. Analysis of the clinical features, serology, and immunogenetics of 100 SLE patients during long-term follow-up. *Q J Med*, **74**: 319–30.

Yokota S (1993). Mixed connective tissue disease in childhood. *Acta Paediatr Jpn*, **35**: 472–9.

5. IDIOPATHIC INFLAMMATORY MYOPATHIES

Agyeman P, Duppenthaler A, Heininger U, Aebi C (2004). Influenza-associated myositis in children. *Infection*, 32: 199–203.

Albani S (1994). Infection and molecular mimicry in autoimmune diseases of childhood. *Clin Exp Rheumatol*, 12(suppl 10): S35–41.

Alexanderson H, Dastmalchi M, Esbjörnsson-Liljedahl M, *et al.* (2007). Benefits of intensive resistance training in patients with chronic polymyositis or dermatomyositis. *Arthritis Rheum*, 57: 768–77.

Antony JH, Procopis PG, Ouvier RA (1979). Benign acute childhood myositis. *Neurology*, 29: 1068–71.

Boulman N, Slobodin G, Rozenbaum M, Rosner I (2005). Calcinosis in rheumatic diseases. *Semin Arthritis Rheum*, 34: 805–12.

Brown VE, Pilkington CA, Feldman BM, Davidson JE; Network for Juvenile Dermatomyositis, Paediatric Rheumatology European Society (PReS) (2006). An international consensus survey of the diagnostic criteria for juvenile dermatomyositis (JDM). *Rheumatology (Oxford)*, 45: 990–3.

Cantarini L, Fioravanti A, Brogna A, *et al.* (2008). Atypical juvenile polymyositis: usefulness of magnetic resonance imaging. *J Clin Rheumatol*, 14: 309–10.

Chan WP, Liu GC (2002). MR imaging of primary skeletal muscle diseases in children. *AJR Am J Roentgenol*, 179: 989–97.

Chevrel G, Calvet A, Belin V, Miossec P (2000). Dermatomyositis associated with the presence of parvovirus B19 DNA in muscle. *Rheumatology (Oxford)*, 39: 1037–9.

Christensen ML, Pachman LM, Schneiderman R *et al.* (1986). Prevalence of Coxsackie B virus antibodies in patients with juvenile dermatomyositis. *Arthritis Rheum*, 29: 1365–70.

Constantin T, Ponyi A, Orbán I *et al.* (2006). National registry of patients with juvenile idiopathic inflammatory myopathies in Hungary – clinical characteristics and disease course of 44 patients with juvenile dermatomyositis. *Autoimmunity*, 39: 223–32.

Dalakas MC (2002). Muscle biopsy findings in inflammatory myopathies. *Rheum Dis Clin North Am*, 28: 779–98.

Dolezalova P, Young SP, Bacon PA, Southwood TR (2003). Nailfold capillary microscopy in healthy children and in childhood rheumatic diseases: a prospective single blind observational study. *Ann Rheum Dis*, 62: 444–9.

Dourmishev AL, Dourmishev LA (1999). Dermatomyositis and drugs. *Adv Exp Med Biol*, 455: 187–91.

Feldman BM, Ayling-Campos A, Luy L, *et al.* (1995). Measuring disability in juvenile dermatomyositis: validity of the childhood health assessment questionnaire. *J Rheumatol*, 22: 326–31.

Feldman BM, Rider LG, Reed AM, Pachman LM (2008). Juvenile dermatomyositis and other idiopathic inflammatory myopathies of childhood. *Lancet*, 371: 2201–12.

Fraser DD, Frank JA, Dalakas M, *et al.* (1991). Magnetic resonance imaging in the idiopathic inflammatory myopathies. *J Rheumatol*, 18: 1693–700.

Gunawardena H, Wedderburn LR, North J, *et al.* (2008). Clinical associations of autoantibodies to a p155/140 kDa doublet protein in juvenile dermato-myositis. *Rheumatology (Oxford)*, 47: 324–8.

Harris-Love MO, Shrader JA, Koziol D, *et al.* (2009). Distribution and severity of weakness among patients with polymyositis, dermatomyositis, and juvenile dermatomyositis. *Rheumatology (Oxford)*, 48: 134–39.

Huang JL (1999). Long-term prognosis of patients with juvenile dermatomyositis initially treated with intravenous methylprednisolone pulse therapy. *Clin Exp Rheumatol*, 17: 621–4.

Huber AM, Feldman BM, Rennebohm RM, *et al.*; Juvenile Dermatomyositis Disease Activity Collaborative Study Group. (2004). Validation and clinical significance of the Childhood Myositis Assessment

Scale for assessment of muscle function in the juvenile idiopathic inflammatory myopathies. *Arthritis Rheum*, **50**: 1595–603.

Huber AM, Lang B, LeBlanc CM, *et al*. (2000). Medium-and long-term functional outcomes in a multicenter cohort of children with juvenile dermatomyositis. *Arthritis Rheum*, **43**: 541–9.

Huber A, Feldman BM (2005). Long-term outcomes in juvenile dermatomyositis: how did we get here and where are we going? *Curr Rheumatol Rep*, **7**: 441–6.

Hundley JL, Carroll CL, Lang W, *et al*. (2006). Cutaneous symptoms of dermatomyositis significantly impact patients' quality of life. *J Am Acad Dermatol*, **54**: 217–20.

Lamminen A, Jääskeläinen J, Rapola J, Suramo I (1988). High-frequency ultrasonography of skeletal muscle in children with neuromuscular disease. *J Ultrasound Med*, **7**: 505–9.

Lewkonia RM, Horne D, Dawood MR (1995). Juvenile dermatomyositis in a child infected with parvovirus B19. *Clin Infect Dis*, **21**: 430–2.

Li CK, Varsani H, Holton JL, *et al*. (2004). Juvenile Dermatomyositis Research Group (UK and Ireland). MHC class I overexpression on muscles in early juvenile dermatomyositis. *J Rheumatol*, **31**: 605–9.

Love LA, Leff RL, Fraser DD, *et al*. (1991). A new approach to the classification of idiopathic inflammatory myopathy: myositis-specific autoantibodies define useful homogenous patient groups. *Medicine (Baltimore)*, **70**: 360–74.

Lovell DJ, Lindsley CB, Rennebohm RM, *et al*. (1999). Development of validated disease activity and damage indices for the juvenile idiopathic inflammatory myopathies. II. The Childhood Myositis Assessment Scale (CMAS): a quantitative tool for the evaluation of muscle function. The Juvenile Dermatomyositis Disease Activity Collaborative Study Group. *Arthritis Rheum*, **42**: 2213–19.

Mackay MT, Kornberg AJ, Shield LK, Dennett X (1999). Benign acute childhood myositis: laboratory and clinical features. *Neurology*, **53**: 2127–31.

Mamyrova G, O'Hanlon TP, Monroe JB, *et al*. (2006). Childhood Myositis Heterogeneity Collaborative Study Group. Immunogenetic risk and protective factors for juvenile dermatomyositis in Caucasians. *Arthritis Rheum*, **54**: 3979–87.

Massa M, Costouros N, Mazzoli F, *et al*. (2002). Self epitopes shared between human skeletal myosin and *Streptococcus pyogenes* M5 protein are targets of immune responses in active juvenile dermatomyositis. *Arthritis Rheum*, **46**: 3015–25.

Miller LC, Michael AF, Kim Y (1987). Childhood dermatomyositis. Clinical course and long-term follow-up. *Clin Pediatr (Phila)*, **26**: 561–6.

Pachman LM, Abbott K, Sinacore JM, *et al*. (2006). Duration of illness is an important variable for untreated children with juvenile dermatomyositis. *J Pediatr*, **148**: 247–53.

Pachman LM, Hayford JR, Chung A, *et al*. (1998). Juvenile dermatomyositis at diagnosis: clinical characteristics of 79 children. *J Rheumatol*, **25**: 1198–204.

Peloro TM, Miller OF, Hahn TF, Newman ED (2001). Juvenile dermatomyositis: a retrospective review of a 30-year experience. *J Am Acad Dermatol*, **45**: 28–34.

Ramanan AV, Campbell-Webster N, Ota S, *et al*. (2005). The effectiveness of treating juvenile dermatomyositis with methotrexate and aggressively tapered corticosteroids. *Arthritis Rheum*, **52**: 3570–8.

Rider LG (2003). Calcinosis in juvenile dermatomyositis: pathogenesis and current therapies. *Pediatr Rheumatol Online J*, **1**: 2 [serial online]. Available at: www.pedrheumonlinejournal.org/march-april03.htm

Rider LG, Miller FW (1997). Classification and treatment of the juvenile idiopathic inflammatory myopathies. *Rheum Dis Clin North Am*, **23**: 619–55.

Rider LG, Miller FW (2000). Idiopathic inflammatory muscle disease: clinical aspects. *Baillieres Best Pract Res Clin Rheumatol*, **14**: 37–54.

Rider LG, Miller FW, Targoff IN, *et al*. (1994). A broadened spectrum of juvenile myositis. Myositis-specific autoantibodies in children. *Arthritis Rheum*, **37**: 1534–8.

Santmyire-Rosenberger B, Dugan EM (2003). Skin involvement in dermatomyositis. *Curr Opin Rheumatol*, **15**: 714–22.

Smith RL, Sundberg J, Shamiyah E, *et al.* (2004). Skin involvement in juvenile dermatomyositis is associated with loss of end row nailfold capillary loops. *J Rheumatol*, **31**: 1644–9.

Summers RM, Brune AM, Choyke PL, *et al.* (1998). Juvenile idiopathic inflammatory myopathy: exercise-induced changes in muscle at short inversion time inversion-recovery MR imaging. *Radiology*, **209**: 191–6.

Taieb A, Guichard C, Salamon R, Maleville J (1985). Prognosis in juvenile dermatopolymyositis: a cooperative retrospective study of 70 cases. *Pediatr Dermatol*, **2**: 275–81.

Targoff IN, Mamyrova G, Trieu EP, *et al.* (2006). Childhood Myositis Heterogeneity Study Group; International Myositis Collaborative Study Groups. A novel autoantibody to a 155-kd protein is associated with dermatomyositis. *Arthritis Rheum*, **54**: 3682–9.

Wedderburn LR, Varsani H, Li CK, *et al.* (2007). UK Juvenile Dermatomyositis Research Group. International consensus on a proposed score system for muscle biopsy evaluation in patients with juvenile dermatomyositis: a tool for potential use in clinical trials. *Arthritis Rheum*, **57**: 1192–201.

Zampieri S, Ghirardello A, Iaccarino L, *et al.* (2006). Polymyositis–dermatomyositis and infections. *Autoimmunity*, **39**: 191–6.

6. VASCULITIS

Akikusa JD, Schneider R, Harvey EA (2007). Clinical features and outcome of pediatric Wegener's granulomatosis. *Arthritis Rheum*, **57**: 837–44.

Benseler SM, Silverman E, Aviv RI, *et al.* (2006). Primary central nervous system vasculitis in children. *Arthritis Rheum*, **54**: 1291–7.

Cakar N, Yalcinkaya F, Duzova A, *et al.* (2008). Takayasu arteritis in children. *J Rheumatol*, **35**: 913–19.

Centers for Disease Control (1990). Revised diagnostic criteria for Kawasaki disease. *MMWR*, **39**(44-13): 27–8.

Dedeoglu F, Sundel RP (2005). Vasculitis in children. *Pediatr Clin North Am*, **52**: 547–75.

Elbers J, Benseler SM (2008). Central nervous system vasculitis in children. *Curr Opin Rheumatol*, **20**: 47–54.

Jennette JC (2002). Implications for pathogenesis of patterns of injury in small- and medium-sized-vessel vasculitis. *Cleve Clin J Med*, **69**(suppl 2): SII33–8.

Kerr GS, Hallahan CW, Giordano J, *et al.* (1994). Takayasu arteritis. *Ann Intern Med*, **120**: 919–29.

Langford CA, Sneller MC, Hallahan CW, *et al.* (1996). Clinical features and therapeutic management of subglottic stenosis in patients with Wegener's granulomatosis. *Arthritis Rheum*, **39**: 1754–60.

Newburger JW, Takahashi M, Gerber MA, *et al.* (2004). Diagnosis, treatment, and long-term management of Kawasaki disease: a statement for health professionals from the Committee on Rheumatic Fever, Endocarditis, and Kawasaki Disease, Council on

Cardiovascular Disease in the Young, American Heart Association. Pediatrics, **114**: 1708–33.

Ozen S, Anton J, Arisoy N, *et al*. (2004). Juvenile polyarteritis: results of a multicenter survey of 110 children. *J Pediatr*, **145**: 517–22.

Phillip R, Luqmani R (2008). Mortality in systemic vasculitis: a systematic review. *Clin Exp Rheumatol*, **26**(5 suppl 51): S94–104.

Saulsbury F (2007). Clinical update: Henoch–Schönlein purpura. *Lancet*, **369**: 976–8.

Saulsbury FT (1999). Henoch–Schönlein purpura in children. Report of 100 patients and review of the literature. *Medicine (Baltimore)*, **78**: 395–409.

Sundel RP (2002). Update on the treatment of Kawasaki disease in childhood. *Curr Opin Rheumatol*, **4**: 474–82.

7. SCLERODERMA IN CHILDREN

Atamas SP, Yurovsky VV, Wise R, *et al*. (1999). Production of type 2 cytokines by CD8+ lung cells is associated with greater decline in pulmonary function in patients with systemic sclerosis. *Arthritis Rheum*, **42**: 1168–78.

Barst RJ, Langleben D, Frost A, *et al*.; for STRIDE-1 Study Group (2004). Sitaxsentan therapy for pulmonary arterial hypertension. *Am J Respir Crit Care Med*, **169**: 441–7.

Black CM (1999). Scleroderma in children. *Adv Exp Med Biol*, **455**: 35–48.

Blaszczyk M, Królicki L, Krasu M, *et al*. (2003). Progressive facial hemiatrophy: central nervous system involvement and relationship with scleroderma en coup de sabre. *J Rheumatol*, **30**: 1997–2004.

Bottoni CR, Reinker KA, Gardner RD, Person DA. (2000). Scleroderma in childhood: a 35-year history of cases and review of the literature. *J Pediatr Orthop*, **20**: 442–9.

Cosnes A, Anglade MC, Revuz J, Radier C (2003). Thirteen-megahertz ultrasound probe: its role in diagnosing localized scleroderma. *Br J Dermatol*, **148**: 724–9.

Cunningham BB, Landells ID, Langman C, *et al*. (1998). Topical calcipotriene for morphea/linear scleroderma. *J Am Acad Dermatol*, **39**(2 Pt 1): 211–15.

Dehen L, Roujeau JC, Cosnes A, Revuz J (1994). Internal involvement in localized scleroderma. *Medicine (Baltimore)*, **73**: 241–45.

DeMarco PJ, Weisman MH, Seibold JR, *et al*. (2002). Predictors and outcomes of scleroderma renal crisis: the high-dose versus low-dose D-penicillamine in early diffuse systemic sclerosis trial. *Arthritis Rheum*, **46**: 2983–9.

Foeldvari I, Zhavania M, Birdi N, *et al*. (2000). Favourable outcome in 135 children with juvenile systemic sclerosis: results of a multi-national survey. *Rheumatology (Oxford)*, **39**: 556–9.

Galie N, Ghofrani HA, Torbicki A, *et al*.; for Sildenafil Use in Pulmonary Arterial Hypertension (SUPER) Study Group

(2005). Sildenafil citrate therapy for pulmonary arterial hypertension. *N Engl J Med*, **353**: 2148–57.

Guariso G, Conte S, Galeazzi F, *et al*. (2007). Esophageal involvement in juvenile localized scleroderma: a pilot study. *Clin Exp Rheumatol*, **25**: 786–9.

Harrington CI, Dunsmore IR (1989). An investigation into the incidence of auto-immune disorders in patients with localized morphoea. *Br J Dermatol*, **120**: 645–8.

Hasegawa M, Sato S, Ihn H, *et al*. (1999). Enhanced production of interleukin-6 (IL-6), oncostatin M and soluble IL-6 receptor by cultured peripheral blood mononuclear cells from patients with systemic sclerosis. *Rheumatology (Oxford)*, **38**: 612–17.

Hoyles RK, Ellis RW, Wellsbury J, *et al*. (2006). A multicenter, prospective, randomized, double-blind, placebo-controlled trial of corticosteroids and intravenous cyclophosphamide followed by oral azathioprine for the treatment of pulmonary fibrosis in scleroderma. *Arthritis Rheum*, **54**: 3962–70.

Jelaska A, Arakawa M, Broketa G, *et al*. (1996). Heterogeneity of collagen synthesis in normal and systemic sclerosis skin fibroblasts. Increased proportion of high collagen-producing cells in systemic sclerosis fibroblasts. *Arthritis Rheum*, **39**: 1338–46.

Jimenez SA, Derk CT (2004). Following the molecular pathways toward an understanding of the pathogenesis of systemic sclerosis. *Ann Intern Med*, **140**: 37–50.

Kähäri VM, Sandberg M, Kalimo H, *et al*. (1988). Identification of fibroblasts responsible for increased collagen production in localized scleroderma by *in situ* hybridization. *J Invest Dermatol*, **90**: 664–70.

Kister I, Inglese M, Laxer RM, Herbert J (2008). Neurologic manifestations of localized scleroderma: a case report and literature review. *Neurology*, **71**: 1538–45.

Koh DM, Hansell DM (2000). Computed tomography of diffuse interstitial lung disease in children. *Clin Radiol*, **55**: 659–67.

Kornreich HK, King KK, Bernstein BH, *et al*. (1977). Scleroderma in childhood. *Arthritis Rheum*, **20**: 343–50.

LeRoy EC, Medsger TA (2001). Criteria for classification of early systemic sclerosis. *J Rheumatol*, **28**: 1573–6.

Li SC, Liebling MS, Haines KA (2007). Ultrasonography is a sensitive tool for monitoring localized scleroderma. *Rheumatology (Oxford)*, **46**: 1316–19.

Liu B, Connolly MK (1998). The pathogenesis of cutaneous fibrosis. *Semin Cutan Med Surg*, **17**: 3–11.

Martini G, Foeldvari I, Russo R, *et al*. (2006). Systemic sclerosis in childhood: clinical and immunological features of 153 patients in an international database. *Arthritis Rheum*, **54**: 3971–8.

Martini G, Murray KJ, Howell KJ, *et al*. (2002). Juvenile-onset localized scleroderma activity detection by infrared thermography. *Rheumatology (Oxford)*, **41**: 1178–82.

Martini G, Vittadello F, Kasapçopur O, *et al*.; Juvenile Scleroderma Working Group of Paediatric Rheumatology European Society (PRES) (2009). Factors affecting survival in juvenile systemic sclerosis. *Rheumatology (Oxford)*, **48**: 119–22.

Mayes MD, Lacey JV, Beebe-Dimmer J, *et al*. (2003). Prevalence, incidence survival and disease characteristics of systemic sclerosis in a large US population. *Arthritis Rheum*, **48**: 2246–55.

Medsger TA Jr. (1994). Epidemiology of systemic sclerosis. *Clin Dermatol*, **12**: 207–16.

Peterson LS, Nelson AM, Su WP, *et al*. (1997). The epidemiology of morphea (localized scleroderma) in Olmsted County 1960–1993. *J Rheumatol*, **24**: 73–80.

Pope JE, Bellamy N, Seibold JR, *et al*. (2001). A randomized, controlled trial of methotrexate versus placebo in early diffuse scleroderma. *Arthritis Rheum*, **44**: 1351–8.

Pope J, Fenlon D, Thompson A, *et al*. (1998). Iloprost and cisaprost for Raynaud's phenomenon in progressive systemic sclerosis. *Cochrane Database of Syst Rev*, **2**: CD000953.

Quartier P, Bonnet D, Fournet JC, *et al*. (2002). Severe cardiac involvement in children with systemic sclerosis and myositis. *J Rheumatol*, **29**: 1767–73.

Rubin LJ, Badesch DB, Barst RJ, *et al*. (2002). Bosentan therapy for pulmonary arterial hypertension. *N Engl J Med*, **346**: 896–903.

Scalapino K, Arkachaisri T, Lucas M, *et al*. (2006). Childhood onset systemic sclerosis: classification, clinical and serologic features, and survival in comparison with adult onset disease. *J Rheumatol*, **33**: 1004–13.

Seely JM, Jones LT, Wallace C, *et al*. (1998). Systemic sclerosis: using high-resolution CT to detect lung disease in children. *AJR Am J Roentgenol*, **170**: 691–7.

Steen VD, Medsger TA Jr (1998). Case–control study of corticosteroids and other drugs that either precipitate or protect from the development of scleroderma renal crisis. *Arthritis Rheum*, **41**: 1613–19.

Tashkin DP, Elashoff R, Clements PJ, *et al*. (2006). Cyclophosphamide versus placebo in scleroderma lung disease. *N Engl J Med*, **354**: 2655–66.

Uziel Y, Feldman BM, Krafchik BR, *et al*. (2000). Methotrexate and corticosteroid therapy for pediatric localized scleroderma. *J Pediatr*, **136**: 91–5.

Weber P, Ganser G, Frosch M, *et al*. (2000). Twenty-four hour intraesophageal pH monitoring in children and adolescents with scleroderma and mixed connective tissue disease. *J Rheumatol*, **27**: 2692–5.

Weibel L, Sampaio MC, Visentin MT, *et al*. (2006). Evaluation of methotrexate and corticosteroids for the treatment of localized scleroderma (morphea) in children. *Br J Dermatol*, **155**: 1013–20.

Zannin ME, Martini G, Athreya BH, *et al*.; Juvenile Scleroderma Working Group of the Pediatric Rheumatology European Society (PRES) (2007). Ocular involvement in children with localised scleroderma: a multi-center study. *Br J Ophthalmol*, **91**: 1311–14.

Zulian, F (2004). Systemic manifestations in localized scleroderma. *Curr Rheumatol Rep*, **6**: 417–24.

Zulian F, Athreya BH, Laxer RM, *et al*. (2006a). Juvenile localized scleroderma: clinical and epidemiological features in 750 children. An international study. *Rheumatology (Oxford)*, **45**: 614–20.

Zulian F, Corona F, Gerloni V, *et al*. (2004). Safety and efficacy of iloprost for the treatment of ischaemic digits in paediatric connective tissue diseases. *Rheumatology (Oxford)*, **43**: 229–33.

Zulian F, Meneghesso D, Grisan E, *et al*. (2007a). A new computerized method for the assessment of skin lesions in localized scleroderma. *Rheumatology (Oxford)*, **46**: 856–60.

Zulian F, Vallongo C, de Oliveira SK, *et al*. (2006b). Congenital localized scleroderma. *J Pediatr*, **149**: 248–51.

Zulian F, Vallongo C, Woo P, *et al*. (2005). Localized scleroderma in childhood is not just a skin disease. *Arthritis Rheum*, **52**: 2873–81.

Zulian F, Woo P, Athreya BH, *et al*. (2007b). The PRES/ACR/EULAR Provisional Classification Criteria for Juvenile Systemic Sclerosis. *Arthritis Rheum*, **57**: 203–12.

8. AUTOINFLAMMATORY DISEASES

Aksentijevich I, Masters SL, Ferguson PJ, *et al*. (2009). An autoinflammatory disease with deficiency of the interleukin-1-receptor antagonist. *N Engl J Med*, **360**:2426–37.

Aksentijevich I, Torosyan Y, Samuels J, *et al*. (1999). Mutation and haplotype studies of familial Mediterranean fever reveal new ancestral relationships and evidence for a high carrier frequency with reduced penetrance in the Askhenazi Jewish population. *Am J Hum Genet*, **64**: 949–62.

Bodar EJ, van der Hilst JC, Drenth JP, *et al*. (2005). Effect of etanercept and anakinra on inflammatory attacks in the hyper-IgD syndrome: introducing a vaccination provocation model. *Neth J Med*, **63**: 260–4.

Chae JJ, Wood G, Masters SL, *et al*. (2006). The B30.2 domain of pyrin, the familial Mediterranean fever protein, interacts directly with caspase-1 to modulate IL-1beta production. *Proc Natl Acad Sci U S A*, **103**: 9982–7.

Drenth JP, Cuisset L, Grateau G, *et al*. (1999). Mutations in the gene encoding mevalonate kinase cause hyper-IgD and periodic fever syndrome. International Hyper-IgD Study Group. *Nat Genet*, **22**: 178–81.

Drewe E, Huggins ML, Morgan AG, *et al*. (2004). Treatment of renal amyloidosis with etanercept in tumour necrosis factor receptor-associated periodic syndrome. *Rheumatology (Oxford)*, **43**: 1405–8.

Federico G, Rigante D, Pugliese AL, *et al*. (2003). Etanercept induces improvement of arthropathy in chronic infantile neurological cutaneous articular (CINCA) syndrome. *Scand J Rheumatol*, **32**: 312–14.

Ferguson PJ, Bing X, Vasef MA, *et al*. (2006). A missense mutation in pstpip2 is associated with the murine autoinflammatory disorder chronic multi-focal osteomyelitis. *Bone*, **38**: 41–7.

Frenkel J, Houten SM, Waterham HR, *et al*. (2001). Clinical and molecular variability in childhood periodic fever with hyperimmunoglobulinaemia D. *Rheumatology (Oxford)*, **40**: 579–84.

Hawkins PN, Lachmann HJ, Aganna E, McDermott MF (2004). Spectrum of clinical features in Muckle–Wells syndrome and response to anakinra. *Arthritis Rheum*, **50**: 607–12.

Hoffman HM, Rosengren S, Boyle DL, *et al*. (2004). Prevention of cold-associated acute inflammation in familial cold autoinflammatory syndrome by interleukin-1 receptor antagonist. *Lancet*, **364**: 1779–85.

Hull KM, Drewe E, Aksentijevich I, *et al*. (2002). The TNF receptor-associated periodic syndrome (TRAPS): emerging concepts of an autoinflammatory disorder. *Medicine (Baltimore)*, **81**: 349–68.

Johnstone RF, Dolen WK, Hoffman HM (2003). A large kindred with familial cold autoinflammatory syndrome. *Ann Allergy Asthma Immunol*, **90**: 233–7.

Kallinich T, Haffner D, Niehues T, *et al*. (2007). Colchicine use in children and adolescents with familial Mediterranean fever: literature review and consensus statement. *Pediatrics*, **119**: e474–83.

Lachmann HJ, Sengül B, Yavuzşen TU, *et al*. (2006). Clinical and subclinical inflammation in patients with familial Mediterranean fever and in heterozygous carriers of MEFV mutations. *Rheumatology (Oxford)*, **45**: 746–50.

Lindor NM, Arsenault TM, Solomon H, *et al*. (1997). A new autosomal dominant disorder or pyogenic sterile arthritis pyoderma gangrenosum, and acne: PAPA syndrome. *Mayo Clin Proc*, **72**: 611–15.

Livneh A, Langevitz P, Zemer D, *et al*. (1996). The changing face of familial Mediterranean fever. *Semin Arthritis Rheum*, **26**: 612–27.

Livneh A, Langevitz P, Zemer D, *et al*. (1997). Criteria for the diagnosis of familial Mediterranean fever. *Arthritis Rheum*, **40**: 1879–85.

Lovell DJ, Bowyer SL, Solinger AM (2005). Interleukin-1 blockade by anakinra improves clinical symptoms in patients with neonatal-onset multisystem inflammatory disease. *Arthritis Rheum*, **52**: 1283–6.

McDermott MF, Aksentijevich I, Galon J, *et al.* (1999). Germline mutations in the extracellular domains of the 55 kDa TNF receptor, TNFR1, define a family of dominantly inherited autoinflammatory syndromes. *Cell*, **97**: 133–44.

Neven B, Callebaut I, Prieur AM, *et al.* (2004). Molecular basis of the spectral expression of CIAS1 mutations associated with phagocytic cell-mediated autoinflammatory disorders CINCA/NOMID, MWS, and FCU. *Blood*, **103**: 2809–15.

Ozen S, Balci B, Ozkara S, *et al.* (2002). Is there a heterozygote advantage for familial Mediterranean fever carriers against tuberculosis infections: speculations remain? *Clin Exp Rheumatol*, **20**(4suppl 26): S57–8.

Ozen S, Ben-Chetrit E, Bakkaloglu A, *et al.* (2001). Polyarteritis nodosa in patients with familial Mediterranean fever (FMF): a concomitant disease or a feature of FMF? *Semin Arthritis Rheum*, **30**: 281–7.

Ozen S, Hoffman HM, Frenkel J, Kastner D (2006). Familial Mediterranean fever (FMF) and beyond: a new horizon. Fourth International Congress on the Systemic Autoinflammatory Diseases held in Bethesda, USA, 6–10 November 2005. *Ann Rheum Dis*, **65**: 961–4.

Prietsch V, Mayatepek E, Krastel H, *et al.* (2003). Mevalonate kinase deficiency: enlarging the clinical and biochemical spectrum. *Pediatrics*, **111**: 258–61.

Reddy S, Jia S, Geoffrey R, *et al.* (2009). An autoinflammatory disease due to homozygous deletion of the IL1RN locus. *N Engl J Med*, **360**: 2438–44.

Rose CD, Martin TM (2005). Caspase recruitment domain 15 mutations and rheumatic diseases. *Curr Opin Rheumatol*, **17**: 579–85.

Saatci U, Ozen S, Ozdemir S, *et al.* (1997). Familial Mediterranean fever in children: report of a large series and discussion of the risk and prognostic factors of amyloidosis. *Eur J Pediatr*, **156**: 619–23.

Samuels J, Ozen S (2006). Familial Mediterranean fever and the other autoinflammatory syndromes: evaluation of the patient with recurrent fever. *Curr Opin Rheumatol*, **18**: 108–17.

Shoham NG, Centola M, Mansfield E, *et al.* (2003). Pyrin binds the PSTPIP1/CD2BP1 protein, defining familial Mediterranean fever and PAPA syndrome as disorders in the same pathway. *Proc Natl Acad Sci U S A*, **100**: 13501–6.

Simon A, Bodar EJ, van der Hilst JC, *et al.* (2004a). Beneficial response to interleukin 1 receptor antagonist in TRAPS. *Am J Med*, **117**: 208–10.

Simon A, Drewe E, van der Meer JW, *et al.* (2004b). Simvastatin treatment for inflammatory attacks of the hyperimmunoglobulinemia D and periodic fever syndrome. *Clin Pharmacol Ther*, **75**: 476–83.

Stojanov S, Kastner DL (2005). Familial autoinflammatory diseases: genetics, pathogenesis and treatment. *Curr Opin Rheumatol*, **17**: 586–99.

Stojanov S, McDermott MF (2005). The tumour necrosis factor receptor-associated periodic syndrome: current concepts. *Expert Rev Mol Med*, **7**: 1–18.

Tunca M, Akar S, Onen F, *et al.* (2005). Familial Mediterranean fever (FMF) in Turkey: results of a nationwide multicenter study. *Medicine (Baltimore)*, **84**: 1–11.

Yilmaz E, Ozen S, Balci B, *et al.* (2001). Mutation frequency of familial Mediterranean fever and evidence for a high carrier rate in the Turkish population. *Eur J Hum Genet*, **9**: 553–5.

Zemer D, Livneh A, Danon YL, *et al.* (1991). Long-term colchicine treatment in children with familial Mediterranean fever. *Arthritis Rheum*, **34**: 973–7.

Abbreviations

AAV	ANCA-associated vasculitide
ACA	anti-centromere antibodies
ACLE	acute cutaneous lupus erythematosus
ACR	American College of Rheumatology
AHA	American Heart Association
ANA	antinuclear antibody
ANCA	anti-neutrophil cytoplasmic antibodies
AoAS	adult-onset ankylosing spondylitis
AP	anterior–posterior (view)
APL	anti-phospholipid
aPTT	activated partial thromboplastin time
ARF	acute rheumatic fever
AS	ankylosing spondylitis
ASO	anti-streptolysin O
BASFI	Bath Ankylosing Spondylitis Functional Index
BCG	Bacillus Calmette–Guérin
BUN	blood urea nitrogen
CAPS	cryopyrin-associated periodic fever syndromes
CARD15	caspase recruitment domain-15
CBC	complete blood count
CCLE	chronic cutaneous lupus erythematosus
CCP	cyclic citrullinated peptide
CHAQ	Childhood Health Assessment Questionnaire
CHB	congenital heart block
CINCA	chronic infantile neurologic cutaneous articular (syndrome)
CLE	cutaneous lupus erythematosus
CMAS	Childhood Myositis Assessment Scale
CNS	central nervous system
CRMO	chronic recurrent multifocal osteomyelitis
CRP	C-reactive protein
CSF	cerebrospinal fluid
CSS	Churg–Strauss syndrome
CT	computed tomography
DIP	distal interphalangeal
DLCO	diffusing capacity of the lung for carbon monoxide
DLE	discoid lupus erythematosus
DMARD	disease-modifying antirheumatic drug
DNase B	deoxyribonuclease B
DPT	diphtheria, pertussis and tetanus
dsDNA	double-stranded DNA
ECDS	*en coup de sabre*
ECG	electrocardiogram
ELE	erysipelas-like erythema
EMG	electromyography
EN	erythema nodosa
EOS	early onset sarcoidosis
ESR	erythrocyte sedimentation rate
ESSG	European Spondyloarthropathy Study Group
FCAS	familial cold autoinflammatory syndrome
FMF	familial Mediterranean fever
GABHS	group A β-hemolytic streptococcal
GER	gastroesophageal reflux
GI	gastrointestinal
GU	genitourinary
HIDS	hyperimmunoglobulenemia D with periodic fever syndrome
HLA	human leukocyte antigen
HLH	hemophagocytic lymphohistiocytosis
HRCT	high-resolution computed tomography
IBD	inflammatory bowel disease
IBP	inflammatory back pain
Ig	immunoglobulin
IL	interleukin
ILAR	International League of Associations for Rheumatology
ISN/RPS	International Society of Nephrology/Renal Pathology Society
IV	intravenous
IVIG	intravenous immunoglobulin

JAS	juvenile ankylosing spondylitis
JDM	juvenile dermatomyositis
JIA	juvenile idiopathic arthritis
JLS	juvenile localized scleroderma
JoAS	juvenile-onset ankylosing spondylitis
JPM	juvenile polymyositis
JPsA	juvenile psoriatic arthritis
JRA	juvenile rheumatoid arthritis
JSpA	juvenile spondyloarthropathy
JSSc	juvenile systemic sclerosis
KD	Kawasaki disease
LE	lupus erythematosus
LSc	localized scleroderma
MAS	macrophage activation syndrome
MCP	metacarpophalangeal
MCTD	mixed connective tissue disease
MEFV	Mediterranean fever (gene)
MMR	measles, mumps, and rubella
MPA	microscopic polyangiitis
MPO	myeloperoxidase
MR	magnetic resonance
MRI	magnetic resonance imaging
MTX	methotrexate
MWS	Muckle–Wells syndrome
NF-κB	nuclear factor kappa B
NK	natural killer
NLS	neonatal lupus syndrome
NOMID	neonatal-onset multisystem inflammatory disease
NSAID	non-steroidal anti-inflammatory drug
OT	occupational therapy (therapist)
PACNS	primary angiitis of the central nervous system

PAN	polyarteritis nodosa
PAPA	pyogenic sterile arthritis, pyoderma gangrenosum, and acne
PET	positron emission tomography
PFAPA	periodic fevers with aphthous stomatitis, pharyngitis, and adenitis
PIP	proximal interphalangeal
PsA	psoriatic arthritis
PSRA	post-streptococcal reactive arthritis
PT	prothrombin time
PTT	partial thromboplastin time
RANTES	regulated on activation, normal T-cell expressed and secreted
ReA	reactive arthritis
RF	rheumatoid factor
RNP	ribonuclear protein
ROM	range of motion
SAA	serum amyloid A
SCLE	subacute cutaneous lupus erythematosus
SI	sacroiliac
SLE	systemic lupus erythematosus
SSc	systemic sclerosis
STIR	short tau inversion recovery (MRI)
TMJ	temporomandibular joint
TNF-α	tumor necrosis factor-α
TRAPS	tumor necrosis factor receptor-associated periodic syndrome
URI	upper respiratory infection
UTI	urinary tract infection
UV	ultraviolet
WBC	white blood cell
WG	Wegener granulomatosis

Index

Note: Page numbers in italic refer to tables or boxes

AAVs, see ANCA-associated vasculitides 114–17
abatacept 27, 34
ACA, see anti-centromere antibodies
acetaminophen 110
Achilles tendon, enthesitis 40
acne, cystic 150
acral blanching 111
acute phase reactants 9
adalimumab 27, 34
American College of Rheumatology (ACR), classification criteria 14, 15
amlodipine 79
amyloidosis 141, 146, 149
ANA, see antinuclear antibody
anakinra 20, 27, 140
ANCA-associated vasculitides 114–17
anemia 72, 128
aneurysm, coronary artery 108
ankle arthritis 21, 52
ankylosing spondylitis, see juvenile ankylosing spondylitis
ankylosis, wrist 32
anti-CCP antibodies 28
anti-CD20 agents 27
anti-centromere antibodies (ACA) 128, 136
anti-deoxynuclease B (DNase B) antibodies 56, 58
anti-dsDNA antibodies 72, 136
anti-IL-1 therapy 146, 147
anti-neutrophil cytoplasmic antibodies (ANCA) 116
anti-streptococcal antibodies 58
anti-streptolysin O antibodies 56, 58
anti-TNF therapy 20, 27, 34, 116, 146, 147, 149
anti-topoisomerase I antibodies 128, 136

antibodies, anti-deoxynuclease B (DNase B) 56, 58
antigenic exposure 38
antimalarial drugs 75, 78–9
antinuclear antibody (ANA) 22, 65, 72, 128, 136
antiphospholipid (APL) antibodies 65, 72, 136
aortitis 118
Arthus reaction 111
atherosclerosis 66
autoamputation 111
autoantibodies
  anti-centromere 128, 136
  anti-DNA 65
  anti-dsDNA 72, 136
  anti-nuclear (ANA) 65, 72
  anti-Sm 65
  anti-SSA 80, 82
  anti-SSB 82
  anti-topoisomerase I 128, 136
  antiphospholipid (APL) 65, 72, 136
  myositis-specific/myositis-associated 97
  RNP 72, 76, 78, 80
  tRNA synthetases 97
autoinflammatory syndromes
  complex genetic 154
  differential diagnosis 142–3
  monogenic 140–53
avascular necrosis 64, 65, 100, 102
azathioprine 79

BABHS, see group A ß-hemolytic streptococcal infections
Baker cyst 22, 23
balanitis, circinate 55
Beau's lines 107
Behçet's syndrome 141, 154
Blau syndrome 150–1
bone inflammation, NOMID/CINCA 145
bone malformations, linear scleroderma 136, 137
bone marrow smear 20

bone scans, systemic JIA 18, 19
bosentan 129
brachial artery, arteritis 119
butterfly rash, see malar rash
buttock pain 38

C-reactive protein (CRP) 9, 19
calcification, soft tissue 98
calcinosis 77, 91, 94–6
calcipotriene 137
calcium channel blockers 79, 129
CAPS, see cryopyrin-associated periodic fever syndrome
CARD15, see caspase recruitment domain-15
cardiac abnormalities
  acute rheumatic fever 56
  JSSc 128
  Kawasaki disease 108
  neonatal lupus 82
  SLE 66
caspase recruitment domain-15 (CARD15) 150
caspase-1 140, 144
CD2-binding protein (CD2BP1) 150
central nervous system (CNS) involvement
  neonatal lupus 81
  primary angiitis 120–1
  SLE 70
cerebral vessels, vasculitis 120, 121
cerebrospinal fluid (CSF) abnormalities 108, 120
cervical spine 16, 17, 28
  facet fusion 28
  polyarthritis 36
  subluxation 28
CHAQ, see Childhood Health Assessment Questionnaire
chest expansion, measurement 44, 45
Childhood Health Assessment Questionnaire (CHAQ) 100
Childhood Myositis Assessment Scale (CMAS) 100

Chlamydia 54
chondrodysplasia, rhizomelic 81
chorea 56
chronic disease
  approach to the child 8–9
  organ involvement 10
chronic infantile neurologic cutaneous articular (CINCA) syndrome *143*, 144–6
chronic recurrent multifocal osteomyelitis (CRMO) 152
Churg–Strauss syndrome (CSS) 114–17
CIASI gene 146
CINCA syndrome, *see* chronic infantile neurologic cutaneous articular (CINCA) syndrome
clavicle, osteomyelitis 152
CLE, *see* cutaneous lupus erythematosus
clinical history 8–9, 10
CMAS, *see* Childhood Myositis Assessment Scale
colchicine 141
cold-induced autoinflammatory syndrome, familial (FCAS) *143*, 144–6
collagen, accumulation in skin 124, 126
complement deficiencies 62, 82
computed tomography (CT)
  angiography 112, 113, 118, 119
  chest 34, 35
  Churg–Strauss syndrome 117
  high-resolution (HRCT) 128
  inflammatory bowel disease 53
  juvenile dermatomyositis 99
  SLE 66, 67
congenital heart block (CHB) 81
conjunctivitis, bulbar 107
connective tissue disease
  decision tree 11
  mixed 76–9
contractures, *see* joint contractures
coronary arteries
  aneurysms 108
  PAN 111, 112
corticosteroids
  CLE 85
  Henoch–Schönlein purpura 110
  intra-articular 34
  juvenile dermatomyositis 100
  localized scleroderma 137
  maternal in neonatal lupus 82

pulse therapy 100, 108
  SLE management 75
  systemic 18, 20, 34
Coxsackie B virus *89*, 103
CRMO, *see* chronic recurrent multifocal osteomyelitis
Crohn's disease 50, 51, 52, 53, 150
cryopyrin 144
cryopyrin-associated periodic fever syndrome (CAPS) *143*, 144–6
cutaneous lupus erythematosus (CLE) 82–5
cyclophosphamide 79, 129
cyclosporine 79
cyclosporine A 20–1
cystic acne 150
cytokines
  cutaneous lupus erythematosus 82
  Kawasaki disease 106
  localized scleroderma 130
  systemic sclerosis 124, *125*
  see also individual cytokines

dactylitis 48, 49
decision trees 11
dermatomyositis
  symptoms 76
  see also juvenile dermatomyositis
desquamation, sheet-like 107
dexamethasone, maternal 82
diagnosis, timeliness 7
digital artery, PAN 111, 113
digital ischemia 79
DIRA, *see* interleukin-1-receptor antagonist, deficiency
discoid lupus erythematosus 83
disease-modifying anti-rheumatic drugs (DMARDs) 26–7, 34
  dosages 26–7
  indications 26–7
  side effects 26–7
  see also named drugs
distal interphalangeal (DIP) joints 48, 49
  distal tuft loss 126, 127
  Gottron papules 92
DMARDs, *see* disease-modifying anti-rheumatic drugs
drugs, in disease etiology 62, 83
dysphagia 76

early onset sarcoidosis (EOS) 150

ECDS, *see en coup de sabre*
echocardiography 19, 108
echovirus *89*
edema
  acute hemorrhagic of infancy 110
  hands 77
  muscle 98
  scrotal 109
en coup de sabre (ECDS) *131*, 134
enteric bacterial infections 54
enthesitis 8, 38, *41*, 54
  hind foot 40
EOS, *see* early onset sarcoidosis
eosinophilic fasciitis 134, 135
erysipelas-like erythema 140, 141
erythema
  annular 80
  cutaneous 71
  erysipelas-like 140, 141
erythema marginatum 56, *56*, 57
erythema nodosa 52
erythrocyte sedimentation rate (ESR) 18, *19*, 96
esophageal abnormalities 136
ESR, *see* erythrocyte sedimentation rate
etanercept *27*, 34, 79, 146, 149
ethnicity 62, 106, 118
etiology, polyarticular JIA 28
etoposide 20
European League Against Rheumatism (EULAR), classification criteria 14, *15*
extension splints 24, 25
eyelid vasculitis 90

face, linear scleroderma 134
familial cold autoinflammatory syndrome (FCAS) *143*, 144–6
familial Mediterranean fever (FMF) 111, 140–2, *142*
fasciitis 134, 135, 149
FCAS, *see* familial cold autoinflammatory syndrome
femoral arteries, arteritis 119
femur, avascular necrosis 65, 100
ferritin 18, *19*
fever
  Kawasaki disease 107, 108
  quotidian 14, 15
  systemic JIA 14, 15, 20
fibrosis, pulmonary 78, 79, 128
fingernails, psoriatic arthritis 49

fingers
flexion contracture 30
tenosynovitis 16, 17
fingertips, pitting 126
flexion contractures 21, 24, 25,
30, 36
FMF, *see* familial Mediterranean
fever
folic acid 100

GABHS, *see* group A ß-hemolytic
streptococcal infections
gastroesophageal reflux (GER)
126, 136
gastrointestinal (GI) disorders 77
Crohn's disease 50, 51, 52, 53,
150
systemic sclerosis 126
gender predilection 21, 106, 124
genetic factors
Kawasaki disease 106
polyarticular JIA 28
SLE 62
geographical variation 42, 118
GER, *see* gastroesophageal reflux
glomerulonephritis 10, 68–9, *68*,
78
glottic stenosis 115
glucocorticoid steroids 18, 20,
100, 137
Gottron papules 92, 93
granuloma
bone 151
cutaneous 150, 151
granzyme A *125*
group A ß-hemolytic streptococcal
(GABHS) infections 56, 58, *59*
growth plates, premature closure
21–2
gums, erythema/telangiectasia 93

hands 16, 17, 32
contractures 36
edema 77
'mechanic's' 92
polyarthritis 30–1
tenosynovitis 16, 17
heart block, congenital 81
heliotrope rash 90
hematologic disorders
juvenile systemic sclerosis 128
Kawasaki disease 107–8
neonatal lupus 80
SLE *65*, 72

hemiparesis 120, 121
hemoglobin levels *19*
Henoch–Schönlein purpura
109–10, 141
hepatic artery, PAN 113
hepatitis B and C infection *89*
HIDS, *see* hyperimmunoglobulinemia D with periodic fever
syndrome
hind foot, enthesitis 40
hip joint arthritis 9, 24, 32, 33, 34
effusions 32, 33
HLA associations
CLE 82
HLA-A2 21
HLA-B8 82
HLA-B27 8, 40, 44, 48
HLA-DQ1 82
HLA-DQ2 82
HLA-DR2 62, 76, 82
HLA-DR3 62, 76, 82
HLA-DR4 76
HLA-DR5 76
HLA-DRw52 82
MCTD 76
oligoarthritis 21
SLE 62
spondyloarthropathies 40, 44, 48
HSP, *see* Henoch–Schönlein
purpura
hydroxychloroquine *75*, 78–9
hyperbilirubinemia 81
hyperimmunoglobulinemia D with
periodic fever syndrome (HIDS)
142, 146–7
hypopyon 39

IBD, *see* inflammatory bowel
disease
IBP, *see* inflammatory back pain
ibuprofen *26*
IL1RN gene 153
ILAR, *see* International League of
Associations for Rheumatology
immunoglobulin G (IgG) 18
immunosuppressive therapy
MCTD 79
SLE *75*
*see also named immunosuppressive
agents*
infectious arthritis 24, 25
infectious disease
associated with Henoch–Schönlein purpura 109

associated with myositis 103
and juvenile dermatomyositis *89*
and PACNS 120
inflammasome 144
inflammatory back pain (IBP) 42
inflammatory bowel disease-associated arthropathy 50–3
inflammatory disease
approach to the child 8
chronic 8–9
see also autoinflammatory
syndromes
infliximab *27*, 34, 79, 108
influenza virus *89*
interferon-ß (IFN-ß) *125*
interferon-γ (IFN- γ) 82, *125*
interleukin receptor antagonists
14, 20, *27*, 140, 146, 147
interleukin-1 (IL-1) 14, *125*
interleukin-1-receptor antagonist,
deficiency (DIRA) 153
interleukin-1, (IL-1,) 144, 146,
150
interleukin-2 (IL-2) 82
interleukin-4 (IL-4) *125*
interleukin-6 (IL-6) 14, 118, *125*
International League of Associations for Rheumatology (ILAR),
classification criteria 14, *15*
interphalangeal joints, psoriatic
arthritis 48, 49
intravenous immunoglobulin
(IVIG) therapy 108
iridocyclitis, *see* uveitis, anterior
IVIG, *see* intravenous
immunoglobulin therapy

Japan 118
JAS, *see* juvenile ankylosing
spondylitis
JIA, *see* juvenile idiopathic arthritis
JLS, *see* juvenile localized
scleroderma
Jo-1 antibodies 97
joint contractures
JSSc 126, 127
management 24, 25
oligoarthritis 24, 25
polyarthritis 30, 36
joint effusions 21
Jones criteria, modified *56*
JSSc, *see* juvenile systemic sclerosis
juvenile ankylosing spondylitis
(JAS) 42–7

juvenile chronic arthritis (JCA),
  classification criteria 14, 15
juvenile dermatomyositis 88–100
  clinical history 89
  differential diagnosis 98–9, 99
  imaging 98
  laboratory testing 96–7
  management 99–100
  physical examination 90–6
  prognosis 99
juvenile idiopathic arthritis (JIA) 8
  classification criteria 14, 15
  clinical history 14–16
  epidemiology and etiology 7, 14
  oligoarthritis 21–7
  polyarthritis 28–36
juvenile localized scleroderma
  (JLS/morphea) 130–7
juvenile psoriatic arthritis (JPsA)
  48–50
juvenile rheumatoid arthritis (JRA)
  classification criteria 14, 15
  pauciarticular (pauci-JRA) 42, 43
juvenile systemic sclerosis (JSSc)
  124–9

Kasukawa criteria 76
Kawasaki disease (KD) 106–8
keloid formation 131
keratoderma blenorrhagicum 54,
  55
keratopathy, band 23, 24
knee
  oligoarthritis 21, 23
  spondyloarthropathy 39
Köbner phenomenon 16
Korea 42

laboratory testing, organ damage
  10
leflunomide 27, 34
leukopenia 65
Libman–Sacks endocarditis 66
limb-length discrepancies 21–2, 23
  management 24
lipodystrophy 96
livedo reticularis 111, 112
liver disease
  neonatal lupus 81
  SLE 66, 67
lupus, neonatal syndrome (NLS)
  80–2
lupus erythematosus, cutaneous
  (CLE) 82–5

lupus nephritis 68–9, 68
lymphadenopathy, Kawasaki
  disease 107
lymphopenia 65

macrophage activation syndrome
  (MAS) 20–1
magnetic resonance imaging
  (MRI)
  juvenile dermatomyositis 98
  polyarthritis 32, 33
  SLE 65, 72
magnetic resonance (MR) angiography 112, 118, 119
Majeed syndrome 152
malar rash 64, 71, 77, 83
MAS, see macrophage activation
  syndrome
MCTD, see mixed connective
  tissue disease
mebendazole 103
mechanic's hands 92
Mediterranean fever (MEFV) gene
  140, 142
meloxicam 26
metacarpophalangeal (MCP) joint,
  psoriatic arthritis 48, 49
methotrexate 20, 26, 79
  dosage 26
  JLS 137
  JSSc 129
  side effects 26
  SLE 75
methylprednisolone 137
  juvenile dermatomyositis 100
  KD 108
  pulsed 108
  systemic JIA 18, 20
mevalonate 146
mevalonic aciduria 146
Mexico 42
microscopic polyangiitis (MPA)
  114–17
mixed connective tissue disease
  76–9
monoarthritis, acute 8
morning stiffness 21
morphea 130–7
  circumscribed 131, 131, 137
  generalized 131, 132
  linear 131, 132, 133–5
  mixed 131
  pansclerotic 131, 134, 135
MPA, see microscopic polyangiitis

Muckle–Wells Syndrome (MWS)
  143, 144–6
mucocutaneous lymph node
  syndrome, see Kawasaki disease
mucositis 52, 107
muscle edema 98
muscle enzymes 96
muscle weakness 96
MVK gene 146, 147
MWS, see Muckle–Wells Syndrome
mycophenolate mofetil 79
Mycoplasma pneumoniae 89
myocarditis 66
myositis, postinfectious 103

nail changes, psoriatic 48, 49
nailfolds, capillary changes 77
naproxen 26
natural killer (NK) cell 125
neonatal lupus syndrome (NLS)
  80–2
neonatal-onset multisystem inflammatory disease (NOMID) 143,
  144–6
nephritis, lupus 68–9, 68, 78
neurologic disease
  mixed connective tissue disease
  76
  PACNS 120–1
  SLE 64, 70
neuropeptides 130
nicardipine 129
nifedipine 79, 129
nodules
  pseudorheumatoid 29
  rheumatoid 29
  subcutaneous 56, 77
NOMID, see neonatal-onset multisystem inflammatory disease
nonsteroidal anti-inflammatory
  drugs (NSAIDs)
  Henoch–Schönlein purpura 110
  oligoarthritis 24
  side effects 24
  systemic JIA 18
nuclear factor-ÍB (NF-ÍB) 150

occupational therapy 34
oligoarthritis 21–7
ophthalmic disease 21
  juvenile idiopathic arthritis 22,
  23, 24, 25
  juvenile localized scleroderma
  136

juvenile spondyloarthropathy 39
Kawasaki disease 107
ophthalmological screening *22*
oral lesions
    IBD-associated arthropathy 52
    Kawasaki disease 107
    ulcers in SLE *64*, *72*, *73*
orbit, pseudotumor 114
organ involvement 10
ossification
    carpal bones 32
    premature 145
osteomyelitis, chronic recurrent
    multifocal (CRMO) 152
osteopenia, periarticular 22, 23, 31

PACNS, *see* primary angiitis of the
    central nervous system
PAN, *see* polyarteritis nodosa
pancytopenia 72
PAPA syndrome, *see* pyogenic
    sterile arthritis, pyoderma
    gangrenosum and acne
    syndrome
parotid swelling 77
Parry–Romberg syndrome *131*,
    134, 135
parvovirus *89*
Patrick test 44
pauciarticular juvenile rheumatoid
    arthritis (pauci-JRA) 42, *43*
PDGF, *see* platelet-derived growth
    factor
penicillin 57, 58–9
pericardial effusion 18, 19, 66
pericarditis 10, 66
periodic fever syndromes 140,
    142–3
petechiae 71
physical therapy 34
PL-12 antibodies 97
platelet counts 18, *19*, *65*, 107
platelet-derived growth factor
    (PDGF) *125*
pleocytosis 108, 120
pleural effusion 10, 18, 19, 66, 67
pleurodynia 103
poikiloderma 96
polyarteritis nodosa (PAN)
    111–13, 141
polyarthritis
    clinical history 28–9
    complications 36
    differential diagnosis 34

epidemiology and etiology 28
examination and diagnosis 32–4
management 34
polymyositis, juvenile 101–2
post-streptococcal reactive arthritis
    (PSRA) 58–9
prednisone
    HSP 110
    JLS 137
    SLE *75*
pregnancy, screening/manage-
    ment of neonatal lupus 82
prevalence 7
primary angiitis of the central
    nervous system (PACNS) 120–1
progressive hemifacial atrophy
    (Parry–Romberg syndrome) *131*,
    134, 135
proline serine threonine phos-
    phatase-interacting protein
    (PSTPIP1) 150
protein:creatinine ratio 72
pseudorheumatoid nodules 29
psoriasis *38*, 48
psoriatic arthritis 48–50
PSRA, *see* post-streptococcal reac-
    tive arthritis
PSTPIP1 gene 150
PSTPIP2 gene 152
pulmonary disorders
    AAVs 116, 117
    MCTD 76, 78
pulmonary embolism 66, 67
pulmonary fibrosis 78, 79, 128
pulmonary hypertension 78, 128
    treatment 129
pulmonary vasculitis 116, 117
'pulseless disease', *see* Takayasu
    arteritis
purpura
    HSP 109, 110
    palpable 109, 110
    SLE 71
pustulosis 152, 153
pyoderma gangrenosum 52, 150
pyogenic sterile arthritis, pyoderma
    gangrenosum and acne (PAPA)
    syndrome *143*, 150–1
pyomyositis 103
pyrin 140, 150

RANTES 118
rashes 10
    heliotrope 90

malar *64*, 71, 77, 83
purpuric 109
raccoon-eye 80
SLE *64*, 71
systemic JIA 14, 16
urticarial 144, 145
Raynaud phenomenon 64, 76, 78,
    94, 124, 126
    management 79, 129
reactive arthropathies 38, 54–5, *55*
    defined 55
    post-streptococcal 58–9
    reactive arthritis (ReA) 54–5
Reiter syndrome 55
renal disease 10
    AAVs 115
    amyloidosis 149
    HSP 110
    PAN 112, 113
    periodic fever syndromes 149
    scleroderma crisis 128
    SLE 10, *64*, 68–9, *68*, *72*, *73*
respiratory disease
    AAVs 116
    JSSc 128
    upper tract infections 56, 58–9,
        109
    see also pulmonary disorders
rheumatic fever, acute (ARF) 56–7
rheumatoid arthritis, *see* juvenile
    rheumatoid arthritis (JRA)
rheumatoid factor (RF) 28, 29,
    128–9, 136, *136*
rheumatoid nodules 29
ribonuclear protein (RNP) anti-
    bodies 72, 76, 78, 80
rituximab *27*, 34, 116

sacroiliac joints
    assessment 44
    inflammatory changes 8, 9, 40, 41
SAPHO syndrome, *see* synovitis,
    acne, pustulosis, hyperostosis and
    osteitis syndrome
'sausage' toe 48, 49
scalp, linear scleroderma 134, 135
Schober test, modified 44, 45
scleroderma *76*, 124–7, 129
    juvenile localized 130–7
    renal crisis 128
scrotum, edema 109
sequelae 7
serositis *64*, 72
shawl sign 90, *91*

shoulder joint 31
sildenafil 129
sinus disease 114
sitaxsentan 129
Sjögren syndrome 77
skin biopsy, JIA 18
skin manifestations 10
    AAVs 115
    cutaneous lupus 83
    HSP 109
    IBD-associated arthropathy 52
    JIA 14, 16
    juvenile dermatomyositis 89,
    90–5
    Kawasaki disease 107
    MCTDs 77
    monogenic autoinflammatory
    syndromes 145, 147, 152, 153
    neonatal lupus 80
    post-streptococcal arthropathy
    56, 57
    psoriasis 48, 49
    reactive arthropathies 54, 55, 58,
    59
    scleroderma 76, 124–7, 129
    SLE 64, 71
skin scoring, computerized 136
SLE, see systemic lupus erythe-
    matosus (SLE)
spinal range of movement (ROM),
    assessment 44–9
splints, leg extension 25
spondyloarthropathy 8, 9
    definition 38
    diagnostic criteria 38
    juvenile 38–42
statins 147
steatohepatitis 66, 67
strawberry tongue 107
strength, assessment 99–100
streptococcal infections
    HSP 109
    myositis 89
    post-infectious arthropathies
    56–9
stroke 70
subdural hemorrhage 70
subglottic stenosis 115, 116
sulfasalazine 26, 34
Sydenham chorea 56
synovial fluid analysis
    JIA 18, 22
    Kawasaki disease 108
synovitis, wrist 9

synovitis, acne, pustulosis, hyper-
    ostosis and osteitis (SAPHO)
    syndrome 152
systemic lupus erythematosus
    (SLE)
    clinical history 64–71
    complications 10, 75
    definition 62
    diagnostic criteria 64–5
    differential diagnosis 72, 73
    epidemiology 62
    etiology 62–3
    imaging 72
    laboratory testing 72
    management 74, 75
    physical examination 71–2
    prognosis 74
    risk of conversion in CLE 84
systemic sclerosis, see juvenile
    systemic sclerosis (JSSc)

Takayasu arteritis (TA) 118–19
telangiectasias, periungual 92
temporomandibular joint (TMJ)
    arthritis 29, 30, 32, 36
tenosynovitis 16, 17
TGF-ß, see transforming growth
    factor-, (TGF-,)
thiabendazole 103
thrombocytopenia 18, 65
tibia
    avascular necrosis 65, 100
    cortical thickening 98
TNFRSF1A gene 148
toes
    arthritis 22
    contractures 36
toxoplasmosis 89
transaminitis 81
transforming growth factor-,
    (TGF-ß) 125
TRAPS, see tumor necrosis factor
    receptor-associated periodic
    syndrome
trauma, as etiological factor 130
triamcinolone hexacetonide 26
trichinosis 103
tuberculous arthritis 24, 25
tumor necrosis factor receptor-
    associated periodic syndrome
    (TRAPS) 143, 148–9
tumor necrosis factor-α (TNF-α)
    125

antagonists/inhibitors 20, 27,
    34, 116, 118, 146, 147, 149
    receptor 148

ulcerations
    mucosal 64, 72, 73
    skin 94
ultrasound
    hip effusion 33, 34
    linear scleroderma 136
upper respiratory infection (URI)
    56, 58–9, 109
urinary tract infections (UTI) 54
urticarial rash 144, 145
uveitis
    anterior 21, 22, 23, 25, 39
    management 26
    posterior 39

varicella 120
vasculitis
    ANCA-associated 114–17
    classification 106, 106
    cutaneous 94, 115
    eyelid 90
    Henoch–Schönlein purpura
    109–10
    Kawasaki disease 106–8
    polyarteritis nodosa 111–13
    primary of CNS (PACNS) 120–1
    Takayasu arteritis 118–19
vasospasm 10
virus infections 89, 103

wall-to-tragus distance 44, 45
weakness
    assessment 99–100
    proximal muscles 96
Wegener granulomatosis 114–17
white blood cell count (WBC) 18,
    19, 65
wrist arthritis 33
    ankylosis 32
    polyarthritis 30
    synovitis 9

xerostomia 77

T - #0379 - 101024 - C176 - 234/156/10 - PB - 9781840761573 - Gloss Lamination